Painless
Evidence-Based
Medicine

Painless Evidence-Based Medicine

Edited by

Antonio L. Dans
Leonila F. Dans
Maria Asuncion A. Silvestre

Asia-Pacific Center for Evidence-Based Medicine
Manila, Philippines

John Wiley & Sons, Ltd

Other Wiley Editorial Offices

John Wiley & Sons Inc., 111 River Street, Hoboken, NJ 07030, USA

Jossey-Bass, 989 Market Street, San Francisco, CA 94103-1741, USA

Wiley-VCH Verlag GmbH, Boschstr. 12, D-69469 Weinheim, Germany

John Wiley & Sons Australia Ltd, 33 Park Road, Milton, Queensland 4064, Australia

John Wiley & Sons (Asia) Pte Ltd, 2 Clementi Loop #02-01, Jin Xing Distripark, Singapore 129809

John Wiley & Sons Canada Ltd, 6045 Freemont Blvd, Mississauga, Ontario, L5R 4J3

Wiley also publishes its books in a variety of electronic formats. Some content that appears in print may
not be available in electronic books.

Library of Congress Cataloging in Publication Data

Painless evidence-based medicine / edited by Antonio L. Dans, Leonila F. Dans,
   Maria Asuncion A. Silvestre ; foreword by Gordon Guyatt.
     p. ; cm.
   Includes bibliographical references.
   ISBN 978-0-470-51939-4 (pbk. : alk. paper)
   1. Evidence-based medicine.   I. Dans, Antonio L.   II. Dans, Leonila F.
   III. Silvestre, Maria Asuncion A.
   [DNLM: 1. Evidence-Based Medicine.   WB 102 P147 2007]
   R723.7.P35 2007
   612.4—dc22

                                2007050370

British Library Cataloguing in Publication Data

A catalogue record for this book is available from the British Library

ISBN 978-0-470-51939-4

Typeset in 10.5/13pt Minion by Integra Software Services Pvt. Ltd, Pondicherry, India
Printed and bound in Great Britain by TJ International Ltd., Padstow, Cornwall
This book is printed on acid-free paper.

Contents

Foreword

No clinician would consider entering clinical practice without knowing the rudiments of history-taking and physical examination. Nor would clinicians consider independent practice without a basic understanding of how the drugs they prescribe act on their patients. Yet, traditionally, clinicians have started practice without an ability to understand evidence about how they should interpret what they find on history and physical examination, or the magnitude of the effects they might expect when they offer patients medication.

Evidence-based medicine (EBM) provides a remedy for this problem. The movement to teach clinicians to become effective users of medical literature began in the 1970s and evolved through the 1980s into a whole system for the delivery of clinical care. We needed a name for this new way of practice and the term 'evidence-based medicine', which first appeared in the medical literature in 1991[1], proved extremely popular. Over the subsequent 16 years evidence-based medicine has evolved and now represents not only an approach to using the medical literature effectively, but a principled guide for the process of clinical decision-making.

Members of the general public are surprised, and often appalled, when they learn that most physicians remain unable to critically read an original research article or fully understand the results reported there. For the physician, inability to critically appraise a research study and grasp all that is implied in its findings limits their independence. The result is reliance on expert opinion, the practices of colleagues and on information from the pharmaceutical industry. But what is one to do if experts and colleagues disagree, or if one is mistrustful of the enthusiastic advice from a pharmaceutical industry representative?

This book represents the key to a world that provides the answer to that question, a world that has traditionally been closed to most practising physicians: the world of original medical literature. Opening the door to this world is enormously empowering. No longer must one choose what to believe on the basis of which recommendation is backed by the most authority, or speaks with the loudest voice. The ability to differentiate high from low quality evidence and large treatment effects from small allows clinicians to make independent judgements about what is best for their patients. It also allows them to explain the impact of alternatives to the patients themselves, and thus to ensure that choices are consistent with patients' underlying values and preferences.

Ten years ago, experts and the official voices of the organizations to which they belonged consistently recommended long-term hormone replacement therapy (HRT) for post-menopausal women. These recommendations were made largely on the basis of observational studies suggesting that women taking HRT could expect large reductions to their risk of major cardiovascular events. Proponents of evidence-based medicine raised concerns about the wisdom of this strong advocacy of therapy for huge populations on the basis of the fundamentally weak methods of observational studies. Their voices were largely ignored, until randomized trials demonstrated that the results of the observational studies were incorrect. If HRT has any impact on cardiovascular disease at all, it is to increase its frequency.

Many clinical communities now endorse widespread population screening to prevent the occurrence of cancer and cardiovascular disease. Breast cancer screening for women as young as 40 years, colon cancer screening for entire populations and treatment to improve lipid profiles even in very low risk patients are widely advocated. Many clinicians are unaware that to prolong a single life, hundreds of individuals must be screened for breast or colon cancer or treated with lipid profile-modifying agents for periods of up to a decade. The costs include anxiety as a result of the many false positive results, complications of invasive procedures such as lumpectomy or colonoscopy, side effects of treatment (including deaths as a result of a lipid-lowering agent now withdrawn from the market) and resource investment that, at least for some individuals, might be better allocated elsewhere. The point is not that the experts were uniformly wrong in suggesting that women consider HRT, nor that screening or treatment of low-risk individuals to modify their cancer or coronary risk is wrong. Rather, it is that clinicians should be aware there are important trade-offs in these decisions. If clinicians don't know the difference between an observational study and a randomized trial, or between a relative risk reduction and a risk difference, they are in no position to understand these trade-offs. If they are unable to understand the trade-offs, it is not possible for them to convey the possible benefits and risks to their patients, many of whom may, with a full understanding, decline screening or treatment.

This book provides the basic tools for the clinician to evaluate the strength of original studies, to understand their results and to apply those results in day-to-day clinical practice. I am delighted to inform the reader that its editors are not only brilliant teachers who have created a wonderful introductory text, but wonderful human beings. I met Tony and Inday Dans just about the time that our McMaster group was realizing that what we had been calling 'critical appraisal' had evolved into a systematic approach to medical practice, a system of thinking about clinical care and clinical decision-making.

Inday and Tony had come to McMaster to train in clinical epidemiology – the science that underlies evidence-based medicine. I had the great pleasure of working with both these brilliant, enthusiastic and critical young people. I was extremely fortunate that Tony chose me as one of his supervisors, and as a result we had the opportunity to work particularly closely together. It was not long before I discovered that I had the privilege of interacting with an extraordinary individual, exceptional even among the lively, intelligent, dedicated students who populated our Masters program. Tony was far more questioning than most students, and possessed a far deeper and more intense social conscience. To me, these qualities were very striking.

Since their days at McMaster, Inday and Tony have continued to demonstrate their high intelligence, tremendous initiative, extraordinary ability to question and explore issues at the deepest level and their unusual and extremely admirable social conscience. Having a social conscience leads you to challenge existing power structures and vested interests. Doing so requires more than conscience: it requires courage. I have had the good fortune and great pleasure to interact with Inday and Tony in a variety of settings at quite regular intervals, and have as a result seen first-hand how their courage has led them to repeatedly challenge authority and power, acting in the interests of the Philippine people. To use the adjective preferred by young Canadians nowadays, their performance has been consistently awesome.

I will add one final anecdote about what makes Tony and Inday so special. Each year, we conduct a 'how to teach evidence-based medicine' workshop at McMaster. In the last few years, Tony and Inday have participated in the workshop in the role of tutor trainees. Almost all participants in the workshop feel they learn a great deal, and take elements of what they have discovered back to their own teaching settings. But very few, and extremely few among the very experienced, make major innovations in their teaching as a result. Despite having run literally dozens of extremely successful workshops in the Philippines prior to their participation in the McMaster workshop, Inday and Tony took the key elements of the McMaster strategy and revamped their approach to their own workshops. The result has been a spectacular success, with Philippine participants reporting profoundly positive educational experiences. In the two decades in which I have participated in our workshop, I've never seen anyone make as good use of their experience with us. The message about Tony and Inday: a tremendous openness and ability to integrate what they've learned and apply in imaginative and perspicacious ways in their own setting.

One fortunate consequence of Inday and Tony's brilliant teaching – which makes the presentation of this book so vividly clear – is that it inspires others. About ten years ago Mianne Silvestre, a neonatologist, attended one of the Dans' workshops and emerged as an EBM enthusiast. She took on a teaching role and emerged as one of the most effective EBM facilitators in the Philippines. Her insights and experience have also contributed to the lucid presentations in this text.

We shall now take advantage of Inday, Tony and Mianne's enormous experience of EBM and their imagination and brilliant teaching abilities in this wonderful book. The title 'Painless EBM' captures the essence of their work. They have presented challenging concepts in simple, clear and extremely appealing ways which make learning EBM painless and enjoyable. They have emphasized the last of the three pillars of the EBM approach: while the book tells you about validity and understanding the results, the focus is on applicability. What is the meaning of the evidence? How can you apply it in your own setting? How can you apply the evidence to patients with very different circumstances and varying values and preferences?

Increasingly, applying the literature to clinical practice does not mean a detailed reading of a large number of original studies. Rather, the clinician can recognize valid pre-appraised resources and differentiate them from poorly substantiated opinion. The book provides guides for assessing not only original studies of diagnosis and therapy, but also systematic reviews which summarize a number of such original studies. The ability to differentiate strong from weak literature reviews and to understand summaries of the magnitude of treatment effects is crucial for efficient evidence-based practice.

When a new pivotal study comes to light, evidence-based clinicians do not need to read it in detail to evaluate its significance or to decide how to use its results. Imagine that I am telling you about a recently conducted study reporting an apparently important treatment effect. I tell you: that the study was a randomized trial and that randomization was adequately concealed; that patients, caregivers and those collecting and adjudicating outcome data were blind to whether patients received treatment or control interventions; that investigators successfully followed all patients who were randomized; and that, in the analysis, all patients were included in the groups to which they were randomized. Assuming that I am skilled in making these judgements, and am telling you the truth, you have all the information you need to judge the validity of the study. If I then provide you with a few crucial details of who was enrolled, how the interventions were administered and the magnitude and precision of estimates of the impact of the intervention on all patient-relevant outcomes, you have everything you need to apply the results in clinical practice.

Synopses of individual studies which provide the crucial information needed to understand the appropriate strength of inference to apply the results are increasingly available, as are systematic reviews and, to a lesser extent, high quality evidence-based practice guidelines. Entire systems of knowledge based on evidence-based principles and textbooks of evidence-based medicine are beginning to arrive. The innovative electronic text UpToDate is an example of a resource that strives to be fully evidence-based and to provide guidance for most dilemmas that clinicians face in practice; UpToDate is effective in meeting both these aims.

When you, as a clinician, have read and digested the current text, you will have the tools to read and interpret synopses and systematic reviews and will be able to find such pearls in the rocky landscape of the current medical literature. In this text you will find case studies and examples directly relevant to your area of clinical practice. More importantly, you will find true-to-life examples of how to address the daily patient dilemmas you face more effectively. You will find clinical practice more satisfying and, most important, you will be more confident in providing your patients with optimal medical care. Finally, if you are interested in a deeper understanding of EBM, this book provides a stepping stone to a more comprehensive text that can provide knowledge and skills required for not only the practice, but also the teaching of EBM[2].

It has been my privilege and joy to reflect on EBM in the context of this wonderful book, prepared by two of my dear friends and their outstanding colleague.

Gordon Guyatt, MD
McMaster University

References

[1] Evidence-Based Medicine Working Group. 1992. Evidence-based medicine. A new approach to teaching the practice of medicine. *Journal of the American Medical Association.* **268**(17): 2420–2425.

[2] Guyatt G and Rennie D (eds.) 2002. *The Users' Guides to the Medical Literature: A Manual for Evidence-Based Clinical Practice.* AMA publications: Chicago, Illinois.

Preface

Inday (Leonila) and I finished our Masters Degrees in Clinical Epidemiology at the McMaster University Medical Center in Ontario in 1991. Since then, our lives have never been the same. The learning culture was unusual at Mac. Education was casual and fun, self-directed and interactive – very different from the serious, didactic, teacher-directed learning that characterized the region where we came from. Distinguished faculty insisted on being called by their first names, rather than 'professor' or 'doctor'. This was difficult for us at first, but soon we began to understand: at Mac, there was only a grey line separating students and teachers.

In the midst of what, for us, was a novel learning environment, we had the great fortune of meeting pioneers in the field of Clinical Epidemiology such as Gordon Guyatt, Brian Haynes, Andy Oxman, Dave Sackett and Peter Tugwell. If there was one thing we brought home from interacting with these professors, it was a passion for lifelong learning. Although the term had not yet been coined, they developed and taught the rudiments of evidence-based medicine: the process of updating one's self to ensure that patients receive not just the latest, but the best medical care.

On our return to the Philippines from the idyllic world of McMaster, we encountered overwhelming obstacles to practising and teaching what we had learned. The infrastructure was not ready for EBM; there was no internet nor e-mail, MEDLINE was not accessible and our medical library at the university seemed like a newspaper stand compared to the library at McMaster. Yes, we worked in an academic setting, but that too was not ready to accept a way of thinking that challenged the *status quo*. Traditional 'experts' felt threatened by EBM, and clinicians were bewildered by the onslaught of alien epidemiologic terms.

To make matters worse, we grappled constantly with the problem of applicability of research conducted in other countries. When are such results applicable to the patients we see? Should we always insist on local studies? What criteria do we use to decide? We had many questions, and hardly any answers. Although the books we brought home from McMaster did not have the solutions, the curiosity we had developed and the creativity we had learned from our mentors there helped us think through the problem. In 1998, with much encouragement and guidance from Gordon Guyatt, we wrote an article on the applicability of clinical trials: our own contribution to the Journal of American Medical Association (JAMA) series of User's Guides to Reading the Medical Literature[1]. Since then, we have developed guides on the applicability of other study designs. We share many of them for the first time in this book.

Another problem which we encountered in trying to teach EBM was the discovery that, unlike healthcare providers in North America, those in developing countries were unable to spare a lot of time reading thick books, listening to long explanations of different concepts of EBM, or attending lengthy workshops or seminars. They didn't want 5-day workshops; they wanted 1-hour lectures. They didn't want a 500-page dissertation; they wanted brief material that could be read in just a few hours. Of course, we insisted on a compromise. Most workshops which we conducted in the 1990s lasted an average of 2 days and the reading material was at least 25 pages. Slowly but surely through these abbreviated meetings, EBM crept into the consciousness of health workers: first among physicians and then among various health-care professionals. These meetings were a tremendous source of gratification, with each workshop bringing new knowledge, new friends and lots of fun.

Dr Mianne Silvestre was one of our participants in these 2-day workshops. Hers is a story we use to inspire other students in EBM. Mianne caught on to EBM really fast. A week after attending her first workshop, she was able to facilitate and teach. A week after that, we heard she had been invited to Singapore to lecture on evidence-based neonatology! This rapid ascent to fame has allowed us to proclaim: you don't need a Masters degree in clinical epidemiology to practice and teach EBM, all you need is a passion for lifelong learning. Her valuable contribution to this book is to ensure that reading it is 'painless'.

With Mianne and eight other enthusiastic participants of our self-learning workshops, we have extended the EBM learning experience through this book. We now provide not 25 but 150 pages of prose, developed through years of trying different approaches to teaching what many consider to be difficult concepts. We have painstakingly put these strategies together to ease the pain of reading and shorten the time it takes to understand EBM. As a result, our publishers have told us that we have an unusually large number of editors and contributors for such a short book. The reason this happened is because we spent years testing the materials on hundreds of workshop participants in the Asia-Pacific region for clarity and re-writing them to make learning exciting and enjoyable.

To augment the simplicity of our prose, we have developed what we call 'tackle boxes'. These are stand-alone tables that help readers grapple with difficult issues without interrupting the train of thought in the text. These tackle boxes come with instructions for use, and often have exercises to reinforce the lessons learned. The result is a simple, concise book which we hope captures the very essence of EBM: lifelong learning that is painless, spontaneous and lots of fun!

We would like to thank Mrs Jemimah Gambito-Esguerra, CEO of the Asia-Pacific Center for EBM, who helped us put together this manuscript; Miguel, our son who, fresh from high school, became our guinea pig to test the manuscript for readability; and Sandra, our daughter, who took time from her studies to draw the cartoons for each chapter.

Special thanks are due to Dr Peter Tugwell and Dr Gord Guyatt, revered mentors and dear friends who inspired us to write this book, and from whom we learned the rudiments of practising and teaching EBM.

Lastly, we thank the thousands of workshop participants in the region whose company we have cherished and who continue to show us how to teach EBM.

Mabuhay!

Antonio L. Dans

References

[1] Dans AL, Dans LF, Guyatt GH and Richardson S for the Evidence-Based Medicine Working Group. 1998. How to Decide on the Applicability of Clinical Trials Results to Your Patient. *Journal of American Medical Association.* **279**(7): 545–549.

List of Contributors

Hilda Diana A. Alava
Department of Pediatrics
Manila Central University FDTMF College of Medicine
Caloocan City, Philippines

Marissa M. Alejandria
Department of Clinical Epidemiology
University of the Philippines College of Medicine
547 Pedro Gil St., Ermita, Manila, Philippines 1000

Antonio L. Dans
Section of Adult Medicine
Department of Medicine
University of the Philippines College of Medicine
547 Pedro Gil St., Ermita, Manila, Philippines 1000

Leonila F. Dans
Department of Pediatrics
Department of Clinical Epidemiology
University of the Philippines College of Medicine
547 Pedro Gil St., Ermita, Manila, Philippines 1000

Aldrin B. Loyola
University of the Philippines College of Medicine
Medical Specialist III
University of the Philippines-Philippine General Hospital
Taft Ave., Manila, Philippines

Jacinto Blas V. Mantaring III
Clinical Associate Professor of Pediatrics
University of the Philippines College of Medicine
547 Pedro Gil St., Ermita, Manila, Philippines 1000

Bernadette A. Tumanan-Mendoza
Institute of Clinical Epidemiology
NIH-University of the Philippines Manila

Benita S. Padilla
Hemodialysis Unit
National Kidney and Transplant Institute
Quezon City, Philippines

Felix Eduardo R. Punzalan
University of the Philippines College of Medicine
547 Pedro Gil St., Ermita, Manila, Philippines 1000

Maria Asuncion A. Silvestre
University of the Philippines College of Medicine
547 Pedro Gil St., Ermita, Manila, Philippines 1000

Maria Vanessa V. Sulit
Asia Pacific Center for Evidence Based Medicine
1344 Taft Ave, Manila, Philippines, 1000

1

Introduction

Antonio L. Dans, Leonila F. Dans, Maria Asuncion A. Silvestre

> *Half of what we learn in medical school is wrong.*
> *We just don't know which half.*

This statement is often heard by freshmen as they are ushered into medical school[1], but it probably rings true for students in nursing, dentistry, midwifery, physical therapy and other allied medical professions as well. A lot of truth dwells in these words. Just a few years ago, we thought that enlarged tonsils had to be removed, pregnant mothers had to be shaved before delivery and vitamin C enhanced immunity to respiratory tract infections. These were non-debatable bits of 'knowledge' then. Today, they are nothing more than sombre testimony to the fallibility of the human mind. Our problem is not healthcare education *per se*. Our problem is progress. Science evolves so fast that what we know now will quickly be outdated if we don't keep up with the literature.

If there was a problem with education in medicine and its allied professions in the last century, it was that professionals

Painless Evidence-Based Medicine   Antonio L. Dans, Leonila F. Dans and Maria Asuncion A. Silvestre
© 2008 John Wiley & Sons, Ltd

were not taught how to keep up with science. We were certainly told that we had to keep up-to-date, but we didn't know how to do this efficiently . . . until 1991. In that year, Dr Gordon Guyatt of McMaster University Medical College in Ontario, Canada, described what he believed were important improvements in the way medicine was taught in his university:

> Clinicians were formerly taught to look to authority (whether a text-book, an expert lecturer, or a local senior physician) to resolve issues of patient management. Evidence-based medicine uses additional strategies, including quickly tracking down publications of studies that are directly relevant to the clinical problem, critically appraising these studies, and applying the results of the best studies to the clinical problem at hand[2].

This is the first use of the term evidence-based medicine (EBM) in published literature. While the emphasis in this passage is on decision-making, the key process has to do with keeping up-to-date with the literature. The faculty of McMaster thought they were on to something exciting[2] – and they were! Within the next few years, the concept spread like fire, becoming one of the most widely-used phrases in the medical literature (see Figure 1.1). EBM was introduced into the curricula of healthcare professionals, first in medicine and later in other fields[3]. Seminars and workshops were conducted across the globe, involving thousands of practitioners from various health care disciplines.

The popularity of EBM is easy to understand. For many the proposed 'rules of evidence' were simple and easy to understand. These rules demystified scientific research, turning it into something busy practitioners could understand, challenge and keep up with. A few 'philosophers' have debated whether EBM deserves the popularity it has gained[4, 5], but the debate has been confusing rather than helpful, fuelled by misconceptions and hurt rather than meaningful differences in opinion. An example of just how confusing the debate has been is as follows:

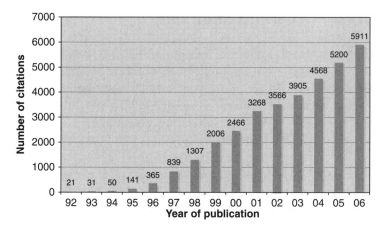

Figure 1.1 MEDLINE citations containing the phrase 'evidence-based' in the title or abstract

The authors reframe the evidence-based medicine debate by pointing out an underappreciated epistemological deficiency: evidence-based medicine as currently conceptualized cannot accommodate concepts that resist quantitative analysis and therefore cannot logically differentiate human beings from complex machines. The authors use Michael Polanyi's philosophy of tacit knowing (which refers to the taken-for-granted knowledge at the periphery of attention that allows persons to understand the world and discern meaning in it) as a starting point for rectifying this deficiency and for working towards an improved, person-centred epistemology of medical practice[6].

We are sure the intellectual ruminations would be fascinating – if only we could understand them. The debate, however, is for philosophers and not for busy healthcare practitioners. For now, all we want to say is this: if you're overwhelmed by the literature in healthcare, then it doesn't matter if you're a physician, dentist, nurse, midwife or therapist, EBM is for you!

1.1   The definition of EBM

Choosing an acceptable definition of EBM is difficult since there are so many definitions available[7]. This is partly because EBM has evolved so much since 1992, and partly because various healthcare professions have modified its definition to suit particular fields. Thus, there are definitions for evidence-based surgery[8], evidence-based nursing[9], evidence-based pediatrics[10], evidence-based psychiatry[11], evidence-based healthcare[12] and even evidence-based alternative medicine[13], to state a few. Our search for the best definition led to the conclusion that there are too many definitions, so what the heck, here's our own:

> *EBM is a systematic approach to the acquisition, appraisal and application of research evidence to guide healthcare decisions.*

Below is our first *tackle box* on understanding the definition of EBM (Tackle Box 1.1). As with other tackle boxes in this book, please spend as much (or as little) time on it as you need to, before proceeding with the text. In the following sections of this chapter, we discuss the three essential skills necessary for the practice of EBM.

1.2   The three skills of EBM

Our proposed definition of EBM requires that healthcare providers demonstrate three major skills to efficiently process the literature. Each skill has several components which are illustrated in Figure 1.2 and discussed in the following sections.

Skill number 1: Acquiring the evidence

The literature on healthcare can be acquired in two modes: by active searching or by browsing[14]. In the active mode, acquisition

Tackle Box 1.1 Components of the definition of evidence-based medicine

Instructions: This tackle box summarizes our definition of EBM and explains various components of the definition. Read column 1 in its entirety before reading the details row by row.

Components of the definition	Explanation of the component
EBM is a systematic approach to the . . .	EBM allows practitioners to assess new (as well as old) technology in an efficient and logical manner, without being intimidated or overwhelmed. This approach requires three sets of skills:
. . . acquisition,	the skill to conduct an efficient literature search and secure a publication in response to information needs;
. . . appraisal	the skill to criticize medical literature and decide if results are credible or not; and
. . . and application of research evidence	the skill to utilize the information in the care of specific persons or populations.
. . . to guide decisions	The evidence itself is only one component of the decisions that need to be made. Other components are tacit knowledge, professional expertise and patients' preferences.
. . . in healthcare.	The skills in EBM have found application in medicine, surgery, physical therapy, nursing, dentistry, primary care, emergency medicine and many other fields including public health.

Note: What have we omitted from other definitions and descriptions?
1. The role of clinical expertise[14]: while this is an important aspect of healthcare decisions, it is a set of skills distinct from EBM, developed and taught in other areas of training of a healthcare professional.
2. The role of patient preferences[14]: again, we feel this is an important element of medical decisions but, like clinical expertise, skills for eliciting patient preferences are distinct from EBM, and are developed and taught in other areas of training.
3. EBM is a philosophy, a movement, or even a scientific revolution[15]. Let's leave the debate to philosophers. This is a book for healthcare practitioners. We say it again - if you are drowning in the medical literature, then EBM is for you!

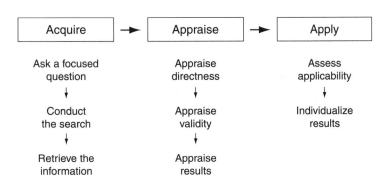

Figure 1.2 The three skills of EBM: how to acquire, appraise and apply the evidence

of evidence is driven by a problem we encounter during the actual care of a specific patient. This triggers a process of search and retrieval for a specific article. In contrast, data acquisition happens by accident in the browse mode, e.g. while leafing through articles in a journal, listening to a lecture series or surfing the net. Most EBM advocates prefer the active mode because the evidence is used almost immediately on a patient. Any lessons learned in this process are more likely to be retained.

Active searches entail three important skills:

(a) how to ask focused clinical questions;

(b) how to search the literature for answers; and

(c) how to retrieve the necessary references.

How to ask focused clinical questions

The most common types of questions asked in clinical practice pertain to the effectiveness of treatment, accuracy of diagnostic tests, prognosis of certain conditions or harmful effects of certain exposures. Whether they are on therapy (Chapter 2), diagnosis

(Chapter 3), harm (Chapter 4) or prognosis (Chapter 5), focused clinical questions have three components: the population of interest (P), the exposure in question (E) and the outcome expected (O). These are explained in detail in their respective chapters. Tackle Box 1.2 includes examples of how to phrase these questions.

Generating focused clinical questions during day-to-day practice is very important because it is during encounters with patients that we come face to face with much of our information needs. Because health technology evolves so rapidly, it is safe to assume that healthcare professionals should be asking these questions all their lives. In an actual healthcare service, this will entail constant vigilance. It will also entail a measure of humility. Instead of posing as professors who know everything, practitioners should role-model curiosity and information-seeking behaviour in their daily practice.

How to search the medical literature

One advantage of phrasing clinical questions as populations (P), exposures (E) and outcomes (O) is that these variables are our gateways to the medical literature. Medical literature databases (such as MEDLINE) usually classify articles according to P, E and O. Looking for articles in these databases becomes a simple matter of using these keywords as filters.

In recent years, managers of these medical literature databases have begun to classify articles according to study design. This is an exciting development because now we can specify not just the topic, but the study design as well.

More details on systematic search strategies are described in the final chapter of this book. It is sufficient to say at this point that the ability to conduct efficient searches is a new skill expected of all healthcare providers. This skill is now a specific expectation in undergraduate and postgraduate curricula for healthcare professionals.

Tackle Box 1.2   Asking a focused clinical question

Instructions: A well-stated question makes it clear whether one is dealing with a query on therapy, diagnosis, harm or prognosis. If the type of question is not clear, then something is wrong. Go through this tackle box to learn the syntax then rehearse the skill while drawing from your own clinical experience.

Type of question	Syntax	Sample question
Therapy	Among P (patients with a certain disease), how effective is E (a certain treatment) in preventing O (an adverse outcome)?	Among children with HIV (P), how effective is isoniazid prophylaxis (E) in preventing tuberculosis (O)?
Diagnosis	Among P (patients with a certain condition), how accurate is E (a certain test), in diagnosing O (a disease)?	Among patients with acute chest pain (P), how accurate is an electrocardiogram (E) in diagnosing acute myocardial infarction (O)?
Harm	Among P (a certain group of patients), how much does E (a potentially harmful exposure), contribute to the causation of O (a certain disease)?	Among healthy males (P), how much does smoking (E) contribute to the causation of lung cancer (O)?
Prognosis	Among P (patients with a certain disease), by how much does E (a prognostic factor), increase the risk of O (a certain complication)? or Among patients with P, how big is the risk of O?	Among patients with prostatic cancer (P), by how much does lumbar metastasis (E) increase 5-year mortality (O)? or Among patients with stage IV breast cancer (P), what is the risk of mortality in the next 5 years (O)?

Note: P = the population of interest (usually characterized by a disease or condition); E = the exposure being evaluated (a treatment, test, harmful exposure or a prognostic factor); O = the outcome expected (a disease, complication or some measure of health). **In a single study, several Ps, Es and Os may be compared at the same time.**

Exercise: Look back to a patient you took care of in the previous week. Think of four focused questions that you could have asked while caring for that patient, and state them in terms of P, E and O.

How to retrieve articles

In most developed countries, once an article has been identified through a systematic search it can almost always be retrieved electronically at the touch of a key. Unfortunately, there are great inequities in access to health information. Libraries in low to middle income countries (LMICs) are generally small and under-resourced. For this reason, journal retrieval can become long-drawn, tedious and frustrating. Methods of tackling this problem include the following:

1. Access free articles online. Many journals such as the Journal of the American Medical Association (JAMA) and Lancet provide free access six to twelve months after publication. Others such as BioMed Central (BMC) are entirely free for the developing world. Freemedicaljournals.com lists journals that currently provide open access. PubMed also highlights such journals. The World Health Organization through the Health InterNetwork Access to Research Initiative (HINARI) provides free online access to major journals to many developing countries.

2. Seek help from multinational companies which have access to extensive library collections (this will be better for your health than seeking free meals).

3. Write to the authors of the publication and request a copy of their article. E-mail addresses are usually listed in the article itself, and authors are often happy to learn of interest in their papers.

4. Keep a list of friends in developed countries, especially those with access to university libraries. Make sure to rotate requests for journals so that they all remain your friends.

If all else fails, you can always pay for online access to an article. The more often you try to retrieve articles, the easier it becomes. Hopefully, one day, someone will address this problem of inequitable access to healthcare information.

Skill number 2: Appraising the evidence

Once an article has been obtained, three aspects of a study need detailed appraisal: directness, validity and results. These are described briefly below, and are discussed in greater detail in Chapters 2–6.

Appraising directness

Directness refers to how well the PEO in the article corresponds to the PEO that you ask. Because medical knowledge is limited, the answers provided in the literature are often similar but not identical. Sometimes the difference is trivial and can be neglected. Other times, however, the differences are important and worrisome.

Appraising validity

Validity refers to how close we think study results are to the truth. As can be seen in later chapters, there are numerous ways in which studies may be flawed. These flaws can lead to biases, meaning they can lead to over- or under-estimates of the things we want to measure such as effectiveness of a treatment, accuracy of a test or causation or prognosis of disease. The higher the number of flaws, the greater is the expectation of bias.

Unfortunately, it is impossible to simply classify evidence as valid or invalid based on study design. The difference between a perfectly valid and a totally invalid study is a huge grey area of intermediate validity. This has led to the concept of a 'hierarchy of evidence', where study designs are ranked according to validity rather than categorized as valid or invalid. The goal of EBM is to identify the best evidence in this hierarchy for each focused clinical question. More will be learnt about evaluating the validity of specific studies in Chapters 2–6.

Appraising the results

We use the term 'results' to refer to numeric expressions of effectiveness, accuracy, causal relationships and prognosis. Examples include the relative risk reduction, number needed to treat, likelihood ratios, odds ratios and hazards ratios. Understanding these numeric expressions can be problematic, especially for the numero-phobic. However, as will be seen, time spent understanding these concepts will eventually be gratified by improvements in the quality of care rendered. We have exerted a lot of effort trying to simplify these concepts in this book.

Skill number 3: Applying the evidence

After acquiring the evidence and appraising directness, validity and results, the last step in processing the evidence is applying it to a particular clinical situation. Two tasks are required: assessment of applicability and individualization of results.

Assessing applicability

Applicability refers to the extent to which conclusions of a study can be expected to hold true for a particular patient. It is similar to directness, but not exactly the same. Directness compares the clinical PEO to the research PEO (in a very general sense). Clinicians can then decide if an article is worth reading or not. Applicability, on the other hand, takes a closer look at specific issues such as biologic and socioeconomic differences between the study population and the patients we see. Clinicians reading articles in scientific journals intuitively ask: will this technology work for my patients? While the hesitation is sometimes well founded, it may actually be unnecessary in some cases. In Chapters 2–6, we share ways of thinking about applicability that have helped us strike a balance between hasty application and excessive caution in the interpretation of results.

Individualizing the results

Studies are concerned with average effects of health technology on large groups of people. As healthcare providers, however, we deal with individual patients whose responses may differ from the average. The estimation of the effect in an individual is therefore an important process. We refer to this process as 'individualization of results'. Individualization is both a science and an art. The science deals with estimation of the magnitude of the effect on a particular individual. This involves some grappling with numbers. The art refers to sharing decisions with patients, laying the cards on the table and using their own values and preferences to assess the trade-offs between benefit, harm and cost.

1.3   Summary

Evidence-based medicine is a systematic approach to the acquisition, appraisal and application of research evidence to guide healthcare decisions. The key skills in EBM help us keep up-to-date with the literature. Acquisition of evidence involves skills in asking focused clinical questions, searching for the evidence and retrieving articles. Appraisal of evidence involves skills in the critical assessment of directness, validity and results. Finally, application of evidence involves skills in the assessment of applicability and individualization of results. Acquisition skills are detailed in Chapter 7 (Literature searches), while appraisal and application skills are discussed more extensively in Chapters 2–6.

References

[1] http://hms.harvard.edu/public/history/past-deans.html; George Packer Berry, 1949–1965. Past Dean of the Harvard Medical School.

[2] Evidence-Based Medicine Working Group. 1992. Evidence-based medicine. A new approach to teaching the practice of medicine. *Journal of the American Medical Association.* **268**(17): 2420–2425.

[3] Green ML. 2000. Evidence-Based Medicine training in graduate medical education: past, present and future. *Journal of Evaluation in Clinical Practice.* **6**(2): 12–138.

[4] Miles A, Charlton B and Bentley P. 2000. New perspectives in evidence-based health care debate. *Journal of Evaluation in Clinical Practice.* **6**(2): 77–84.

[5] Miles A, Bentley P, Polychronis A and Grey J. 1997. Evidence-based Medicine: Why all the fuss? This is why. *Journal of Evaluation in Clinical Practice.* **3**(2): 83–86.

[6] Henry SG, Zaner RM and Dittus R. 2007. Viewpoint: Moving beyond Evidence-based Medicine. *Academy of Medicine.* **82**(3): 292–297.

[7] Beutow S and Kenealy T. 2000. Evidence Based Medicine: need for new definition. *Journal of Evaluation in Clinical Practice.* **6**(2): 85–92.

[8] Toledo-Pereyra LH. 2005. Evidence-Based Surgery. *Journal of Investigative Surgery.* **18**(5): 219–222.

[9] DiCenso A, Cullum N and Ciliska D. 1998. Implementing evidence-based nursing: some misconceptions [editorial]. *Evidence-Based Nursing.* **1**: 38–40.

[10] Moyer VA and Elliott EJ. 2000. Preface *In* Moyer VA, Elliott EJ, Davis RL, Gilbert R, Klassen T, Logan S, Mellis C and Williams K (eds.). *Evidence based pediatrics and child health.* London: BMJ Books.

[11] Goldbloom DS. 2003. Evidence-based psychiatry [editorial]. *CPA Bulletin.* **35**(6): 3, 5.

[12] Hicks N. 1997. Evidence based healthcare. *Bandolier.* **4**(39): 8. http://www.jr2.ox.ac.uk/bandolier/band39/b39-9.html

[13] Mills EJ, Hollyer T, Guyatt G, Ross CP, Saranchuk R and Wilson K. 2002. Evidence-Based Complementary and Alternative Medicine Working Group. Teaching evidence-based complementary and alternative medicine: 1. A learning structure for clinical decision changes. *Journal of Alternative Complementary Medicine.* **8**(2): 207–214.

[14] Sackett, D. 2000. *Evidence-based Medicine: How to Practice and Teach EBM.* 2nd edition. Churchill Livingstone.

[15] Seton SR and Stanley DE. 2003. A philosophical analysis of the evidence-based medicine debate. *BMC Health Services Research.* **3**: 14.

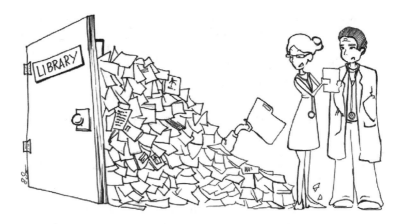

Good! You acquired the article! Now you need to appraise and apply.

2

Evaluation of Articles on Therapy

Leonila F. Dans, Hilda Diana A. Alava, Antonio L. Dans, Benita S. Padilla

Questions on effectiveness of therapy should be phrased in terms of the variables: P, the patient population with a certain disease or condition; E, the exposures (or treatments) to be administered to these patients; and O, the outcomes (or conditions) that the treatments are intended to prevent or promote. For example:

> Among children 1–5 years of age (P), how effective is zinc supplementation compared to placebo (E), in preventing acute diarrhoea (O)?

As can be seen in this example, there are usually two exposures in a therapy question: the experimental treatment being evaluated (usually a new one) and the control therapy to which it is being compared. The control therapy can be a *neutral* control with no expected effect (e.g. a placebo), or an *active* control which constitutes what is considered the most effective treatment at the time of investigation.

Painless Evidence-Based Medicine   Antonio L. Dans, Leonila F. Dans and Maria Asuncion A. Silvestre
© 2008 John Wiley & Sons, Ltd

Outcomes in each of these treatment groups are compared in therapy trials. Some outcomes are *dichotomous*, meaning there are only two possible results, e.g. death or survival. Dichotomous outcomes are usually summarized as proportions (e.g. the proportion that died in each treatment group). Other outcomes are *continuous* in nature, meaning there is a wide range of possible results (e.g. changes in weight). Continuous outcomes are commonly summarized as means (e.g. the mean change in weight in each treatment group).

2.1 Appraising directness

Before even reading an article, the first thing we must do is evaluate *directness*, i.e. how well the PEO in the study (the research question), corresponds with our own PEO (the clinical question). The problem of directness is very common. Directness issues arise because investigators are constrained by their budgets to answer very narrow, focused questions. In contrast, healthcare professionals in the real world are interested in a very broad range of issues. These differences are summarized in Table 2.1.

Because the evidence doesn't always provide a direct answer to our clinical question, we are often constrained to use available information. For example, we have used studies in men to manage coronary disease in women for many decades[1]. Also, few beta-blockers have been proven to reduce the risk of stroke in hypertensive patients and yet specialty societies agree that any beta-blocker may be used[2].

There are instances however, when we should be very cautious in using indirect evidence. For example, a study on the anti-arrhythmic drug flecainide for acute myocardial infarction (MI)[3] showed that, despite the beneficial effect on cardiac rhythm (the surrogate outcome), the drug eventually caused thousands of

Table 2.1 The problem of directness: differences in the types of questions asked by researchers and clinicians according to the population of interest (P), the exposures or treatments evaluated (E) and the outcomes monitored (O)

	Research Questions	Clinical Questions
P	Because sample size is limited, researchers need to restrict their studies to a few, broadly defined subgroups of patients e.g. the effect of treatment in the young and old.	Clinically, we are often interested in treatment effects in many different subgroups e.g. the effect of treatment in young and old, males and females, sick and healthy, smokers and non-smokers, rich and poor.
E	Researchers usually evaluate a specific exposure e.g. drug preparation, surgical technique or educational strategy.	Clinically, we are usually interested in variations of the exposure e.g. a similar drug belonging to the same class, a similar surgery using a modified technique, or a similar educational strategy using a different educational tool.
	Researchers sometimes make inappropriate comparisons e.g. a high dose of one drug *versus* a low dose of another.	Clinically, we are only interested in fair comparisons.
O	Researchers usually monitor a selected few, easily measurable outcomes e.g. surrogate outcomes such as serum cholesterol and blood pressure.	Clinically, we are more interested in important effects that are sometimes difficult and expensive to measure e.g. clinical outcomes such as pain relief, disability, overall quality of life or mortality.
	Researchers at times monitor composite outcomes e.g. instead of measuring the incidence of death alone, they monitor the combined incidence of death, stroke or heart attack. This increases the number of events in a study, and thus decreases the required sample size.	Clinically, we are interested in the effect of treatment on separate outcomes because in composite outcomes 1) the individual components may not be of equal importance to us or 2) the effect of treatment may not be of the same magnitude for each component.

deaths in the setting of an acute MI (the clinical outcome)[4]. If we are to avoid harming patients the way this drug did, we must think twice before assuming that a surrogate outcome, such as reducing cardiac rhythm problems, provides a direct answer to a clinically important question, such as prolonging life.

Evaluating directness is as much an art as it is a science. If you feel the article might provide a reasonably close answer to the question you are asking, then proceed to evaluate it in greater detail. Otherwise, it would be wise to spend your time looking for a closer match.

2.2   Appraising validity

The validity of trials comparing two therapies depends almost entirely on how fair the comparisons are between patients in the treatment and control groups. We summarize eight criteria for assessing validity. These criteria are phrased as questions. A 'yes' answer to a question means that the criterion is satisfied. The more 'yes' answers there are, the more sure we become that the comparisons are fair and that the odds are not stacked in favour of one group (a phenomenon known as *bias*).

Question 1: Were patients randomly assigned to treatment groups?

Random assignment of patients to treatment groups in a trial is the best technique to ensure that treatment groups are truly comparable. If patients are not assigned to treatment groups at random, then allocation may become unfair. Cases with poorer prognosis may end up being assigned to one treatment group.

Historically, a coin toss could be used to assign patients to either treatment group. More frequently, tables of random numbers and, more recently, computer-generated random sequences have been used.

Studies that use this strategy to compare two treatments are referred to as randomized controlled trials (RCTs). Such trials are considered the highest form of evidence on therapy. However, there are some situations where we cannot insist on randomization. For example, when one therapy is clearly superior to another in reversing the course of a disease, it would be unethical to conduct an RCT. In such situations (e.g. blood transfusion for massive haemorrhage, or surgical repair of perforating abdominal injuries), we can usually assume effectiveness. Unfortunately, such miracle cures are the exception rather than the rule. In general, we search for RCTs before accepting a claim that a therapy is effective.

Tip: To check if randomization was performed, look for the words 'randomization', 'randomized' or 'randomly allocated/ assigned' in the title, abstract or methodology.

Question #2: Was allocation concealed?

In a trial, the random order by which we assign patients to treatment groups is referred to as the allocation sequence. It is not sufficient that researchers generate an allocation sequence that is random; they must also take measures to ensure that the sequence is not altered by clinicians who unknowingly (or knowingly) tend to disturb it. These measures are called allocation concealment strategies. One such measure is placement of treatment assignments in sealed opaque envelopes. Other investigators assign a third party not involved in the study (e.g. a pharmacist) to assign the treatment. More recently, objective computers have replaced subjective humans in the task of allocating treatment.

Tip: To ascertain allocation concealment, look for a phrase or paragraph stating one of the following:

1. that a clinician recruiting a patient must contact a remote centre to obtain a patient treatment assignment;

2. that envelopes containing the allocation sequence were sealed and numbered; or

3. that vehicles or packages containing the medications were indistinguishable.

Question #3: Were baseline characteristics similar at the start of the trial?

Because of randomization, baseline characteristics of treatment groups in an RCT tend to be *very* similar. Sometimes, however, inequality between treatment groups may arise due to chance alone. This third criterion checks how successful randomization and allocation concealment were by actually comparing the characteristics of patients within the treatment and control groups.

The comparisons are usually presented as a table of baseline characteristics with columns for treatment and control groups. Sometimes there is also a column of p-values but this is not as important. A p-value just tells us if the difference occurred by chance. What we really need to know is if the difference is big enough to affect the results by putting one group at a disadvantage. Thus, when studies report, 'There was no statistically significant difference between the two groups for baseline characteristics', try to assess if the magnitude of the differences are *clinically* important. For example, a difference in mean gestational age of 31 weeks *versus* 33 weeks among premature babies may be statistically insignificant (p > 0.05). However, this difference may still be clinically important in a trial assessing a therapy to prevent hyaline membrane disease.

Question #4: Were patients blinded to treatment assignment?

If patients know which treatment they are receiving (active drug or placebo), they can subconsciously or even deliberately influence their own outcomes. This may occur, especially when the outcomes being monitored are subjective. For example, there may be a tendency to report symptoms if they know they are taking placebo. This will make the active drug seem better.

Tip: To decide if patients were blinded during conduct of the trial, look for use of identical preparations. Obviously, blinding is more difficult (even impossible) when the interventions involve diet, educational manoeuvres or surgical procedures.

Do not confuse blinding with allocation concealment. Blinding is an attempt to make the treatments being compared indistinguishable. In contrast, allocation concealment is an attempt to preserve the allocation sequence (as described in Question #2 above).

Question #5: Were caregivers blinded to treatment assignment?

When caregivers and physicians are aware of the treatment group to which patients are assigned, they may treat the patients in the two groups differently. For example, a clinician who knows his patient is on a placebo may worry and decide to take better care of that patient. Conversely, a clinician who knows the patient is on treatment may decide to monitor more frequently just in case there are side effects. These changes in care may make a treatment appear better or worse than it really is.

Tip: To decide if caregivers were blinded in the conduct of the trial, look for use of identical preparations. Again, blinding is not always possible. It can be very difficult when the interventions involve diet, educational manoeuvres, or surgical procedures.

Question #6: Were outcome assessors blinded to treatment assignment?

Outcome assessors can be the patients themselves, or their caregivers. They are sometimes directly involved in assessing outcomes or therapy response. For example, patients may be asked if they feel better and caregivers may be asked if they think their patients are doing well. The potential bias involved in this task can often be reduced by blinding them to treatment assignments as described in Questions #4 and #5.

Sometimes, however, the outcome assessors are study personnel (for example, members of an endpoint committee), responsible for deciding how a patient responded to therapy. The questions these personnel answer can become very tricky. Was this hospitalization a result of a drug side effect? Did this patient die of a heart attack or pneumonia? Is this rise in creatinine significant or not?

Because their decisions are often subjective, information on treatment assignment should be withheld from outcome assessors whenever they review a case. This is an important strategy. As mentioned in Questions #4 and #5, blinding of patients and their caregivers may be difficult or impossible in some trials. However, blinding study personnel when they assess outcomes is almost always doable (with rare exceptions). This will usually ensure a more objective evaluation.

Tip: First decide who is making the outcome assessment: the patient, the caregiver or the investigator. If it is the patient or caregiver, tips to answer Questions #5 and #6 will apply. If it is the investigator, look for statements indicating that they were 'blinded', that clinical data was withheld, or that their assessments were independent.

Question #7: Were all patients analysed in the groups to which they were originally randomized?

As in the real world, patients in trials may not comply or adhere to the treatment protocol that they were assigned to. This may happen for many reasons. They may forget how to take a drug properly, suffer intolerable side effects, or even refuse to go on for no apparent reason. A dilemma arises: should they be analysed in their original treatment group (intention-to-treat analysis), or should they just be excluded from the study (censored analysis)?

There are two reasons why non-compliant patients should be analysed in their original groups. Firstly, in the real world, a patient's ability to comply is considered part of the performance (success or failure) of that therapy. If investigators remove non-compliant patients from their analysis, the treatments may appear better than they actually are. Secondly, non-compliant patients should be analysed in their original assignments because removing them could disturb the balance achieved by random allocation.

Tip: To make sure that investigators did not censor non-compliant patients from the analysis, look for the term 'intention-to-treat' under the analysis section of the article. If not stated explicitly, look for some indication that patients retained their original assignment even if they were non-compliant. If this is not stated as well, a last resort would be to check that the number of patients randomized is equal to the number of patients analysed at the end of the study. This suggests (but does not guarantee) that patients were not excluded from the analysis.

Question #8: Was follow-up rate adequate?

Adequacy of follow-up refers to minimization of the number of patients who drop out from a study. Drop-outs are not the same as non-compliant patients (discussed in Question #7 above). Non-compliant patients stop taking the drug, but we can still determine what happened to them. In fact, as previously discussed, we can still include them in the analysis. In contrast, drop-outs leave the study (or are removed), leaving us with no data on their outcomes. Drop-outs usually leave the study because of adverse events or dissatisfaction. The greater the number of patients lost to follow-up, the more the study validity is threatened. The crucial issue is ascertaining when to worry about the number of drop-outs. Tackle Box 2.1 provides an approach to this problem. Essentially, readers should worry about drop-out rates when they are large enough to affect the outcome of a trial.

The eight questions on the validity of a study have now been discussed. While it is tempting to be strict and insist that all eight criteria be satisfied, we must be pragmatic and remember that we sometimes need to make medical decisions based on less than perfect information. If you feel that errors are small or that this is probably the best study you will find that addresses your clinical question, read the results. If you feel the errors are too great and that there are better studies, then don't waste your time with the article.

2.3   Appraising the results

Question #1: How large was the effect of treatment?

The magnitude of the treatment effect may be expressed by comparing outcomes in the treatment and control groups. As described earlier, outcomes can be reported either as:

1. continuous variables, which have a range of possible results (e.g. change in weight, or change in quality of life on a scale of zero to one); or

2. dichotomous variables, which have only one of two possible results (e.g. dead or alive, hospitalized or not).

When the outcomes are continuous, the effect of treatment is simply expressed as the 'mean difference'. This is easily calculated by obtaining the mean result in the treatment and control groups and calculating the difference, that is

Mean difference = *mean in control group* − *mean in treatment group.*

For example, if a trial on hypertension showed the mean systolic blood pressure in the control to be 160 mmHg and the mean in the treatment group to be 120 mmHg, then the mean difference would be 40 mmHg.

Unfortunately, things are not as straightforward when dealing with dichotomous outcomes. Tackle Box 2.2 attempts to simplify this task. If unfamiliar with the concepts of relative risk reduction, absolute risk reduction and relative risk, take time to study this box. If you have heard of these concepts but have difficulty remembering them, the box provides some tricks to help you recall them in an instant.

Tackle Box 2.1 Assessing if there are too many drop-outs in a study

Instructions: In this hypothetical RCT, patients with severe pneumonia are randomized to receive either active treatment (n = 30) or placebo (n = 30). There are 13 drop-outs in the study, 6 on treatment and 7 on placebo. Go through this tackle box by rows to learn how to decide if there are too many drop-outs in a study.

	Treatment group N = 30	Placebo group N = 30
Step 1: Count the number of patients with bad outcomes in each treatment group, and express this as a fraction of the number of patients analysed	Deaths $= \dfrac{5}{24}$	Deaths $= \dfrac{9}{23}$
Step 2: Count the number of drop-outs in each treatment group	Drop-outs $= 6$	Drop-outs $= 7$
Step 3: Create a *worst* scenario for the treatment group by assuming all the drop-outs in this group had the bad outcome, and all the drop-outs in the control group had a good outcome	Deaths $= \dfrac{5+6}{24+6} = \dfrac{11}{30}$	Deaths $= \dfrac{9+0}{23+7} = \dfrac{9}{30}$

Step 4: Create a best scenario for the treatment group by assuming the opposite, i.e. all the drop-outs in this group had a good outcome, and all the drop-outs in the control group had the bad outcome	Deaths $= \dfrac{5+0}{24+6} = \dfrac{5}{30}$	Deaths $= \dfrac{9+7}{23+7} = \dfrac{16}{30}$
Step 5: Were the conclusions of the best and worst scenarios significantly different? If yes, then there were too many drop-outs!	The best-case scenario showed fewer bad events for treatment (benefit), while the worst-case scenario showed more bad events for treatment (harm). Therefore, there were too many drop-outs in this hypothetical study.	

Note – This process of making best and worst assumptions about what happened to drop-outs is called a sensitivity analysis. In essence, we are trying to find out if the conclusions are sensitive to the assumptions we make. If it didn't matter what happened to the drop-outs, we say the conclusions are 'robust'. If what happened to the drop-outs will significantly change our conclusions, however, we say that the conclusions are 'soft'.

Exercise – If the deaths on treatment were 1/24 and the deaths on placebo were 16/23, would the same drop-out rates still be worrisome? (Answers: No, the treatment group would have fewer deaths in both the best and worst scenarios.)

Tackle Box 2.2 Measures of effectiveness for dichotomous outcomes

Instructions: Before going through this tackle box, imagine you went on a diet and lost weight from 80 kg to 60 kg. Now spend a few minutes to think of different ways of numerically expressing your weight loss. We've listed some ways to do this in column 1. Start by going through this column, then through columns 2–5, to understand different measures of effectiveness.

Weight analogy		Measures of effectiveness		
In what ways could you express your change in weight if it went down from 80 kg (W_c) to 60 kg (W_t)?	What subliminal formula did you use to come up with these expressions?	Similarly, in what ways could you express a change in the risk of death from 8% in a control group (R_c) to 6% in a treatment group (R_t)?	What would the formulae be for these expressions?	How would you interpret these numbers?
'I lost 25% of my weight' – your relative weight reduction.	$\dfrac{\text{weight change}}{\text{original weight}} = \dfrac{W_c - W_t}{W_c}$	'I lost 25% of my risk'. This is called the relative risk reduction or RRR, and it is usually expressed in %.	$RRR = \dfrac{\text{risk change}}{\text{original risk}} = \dfrac{R_c - R_t}{R_c}$	RRR (usually in percent): >0% Treatment beneficial ~0% Treatment no effect <0% Treatment harmful
'I lost 20 kg' – your absolute weight reduction.	weight change $= W_c - W_t$	'I lost 2% of my risk'. This is called the absolute risk reduction or ARR, and it is usually expressed in %.	$ARR = \text{risk change}$ $= R_c - R_t$ $= 8\% - 6\%$	ARR (usually in percent): >0% Treatment beneficial ~0% Treatment no effect <0% Treatment harmful
'I now weigh 75% of what I used to weigh' – your relative weight.	$\dfrac{\text{new weight}}{\text{original weight}} = \dfrac{W_t}{W_c}$	'My risk is now 0.75 of what it was'. This is called the relative risk or RR, and it is usually expressed as a decimal number.	$RR = \dfrac{\text{new risk}}{\text{original risk}} = \dfrac{R_t}{R_c}$ $= \dfrac{6}{8}$	RR (usually in decimals): <1.0 Treatment beneficial ~1.0 Treatment no effect >1.0 Treatment harmful

Notes:

1) Look at the middle column. One statement reads 'I lost 25% of my risk'. The other statement reads 'I lost 2% of my risk'. Can both of these statements be correct, given the same data? The answer is yes. Note however, that the first is a relative reduction and the second an absolute reduction. Authors like to report relative reductions because they are constant and they also seem bigger. Readers should also look for the absolute reductions.

2) Look at the last column. These interpretations of ARR, RRR and RR assume that the outcomes are reported as **unfavourable** events (e.g. death), rather than favourable events (e.g. survival). If the outcome is reported as the proportion that survived instead of the proportion that died, all the interpretations are reversed. An RRR >0% could actually mean harm instead of benefit. We think authors should always report the harmful outcome to avoid confusion. Also, we feel that it sounds really pessimistic to report 'the relative risk of surviving'. Unfortunately, not everyone agrees.

3) Aside from the RRR, ARR and RR, there is a fourth measure of treatment effects not shown in the table. This is known as the number needed to treat, or NNT. This is derived from the ARR. In the example above, the ARR is 2%, which means 'I can prevent 2 deaths out of every 100 patients that I treat'. Thus, I need to treat 50 patients before I save one life. NNT, therefore, is simply calculated as 100/ARR (since it is reported in percent). It tells us the number of patients we would need to treat to prevent 1 adverse outcome. The closer the NNT is to one, the more effective the treatment. The higher it is above one, the less effective the treatment is. When the ARR is <0 (i.e. when treatment is harmful), NNT will also be negative. In this situation it is sometimes referred to as the number needed to *harm* (NNH).

Exercise:

1. If an RCT showed death rates of 4% in the treatment group and 5% in the placebo group, what would the RRR, ARR, RR and NNT be?
2. What if death rates were 5% on treatment and 4% on placebo?

Answers: 1. RRR = 20%, ARR = 1%, RR = 0.80, NNT = 100; 2. RRR = −25%, ARR = −1%, NNH = 100.

Another way of summarizing dichotomous outcomes is by using rates instead of proportions. As the term suggests, rates tell us how fast events accumulate in treatment and control groups through time. Thus, if a clinical trial is conducted over a four-year period, the results can be stated as either: 40% of patients died in the control group and 20% in treatment (proportions); or 10% died per year in the control group, and 5% died per year in the treatment group (rates). The difference can be graphically illustrated in *survival curves* as shown in Figure 2.1.

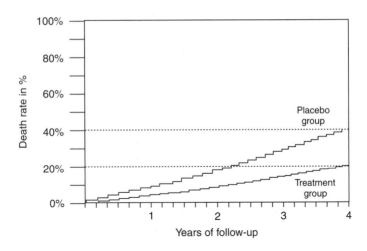

Figure 2.1 Survival curve of a hypothetical randomized controlled trial

A common expression comparing two rates would be the hazards ratio, which is the rate of outcomes on treatment divided by the rate of outcomes in control. This expression is similar to the relative risk (RR). It is interpreted in exactly the same way and it is usually different by just a few decimal places. The various ways of expressing effectiveness are summarized in Table 2.2 below.

Table 2.2   Ways of expressing effectiveness

Outcome	Summary of result within each group	Comparison of results between two groups
Dichotomous (e.g. lived or died, BP controlled or not)	Proportion (e.g. deaths per 100 patients)	Relative risk reduction, absolute risk reduction, relative risk (see Tackle Box 2.2)
	Rate = e.g. deaths per 100 patients per year	Hazard ratio = rate in treatment/rate in control group
Continuous (e.g. blood pressure in mmHg, quality of life on a scale of 0 to 1)	Mean (e.g. mean blood pressure)	Mean difference = mean in control − mean in treatment group

Question #2: How precise was the estimate of the treatment effect?

Because a study merely estimates the true effect of a drug, it may be unduly confident to express absolute risk reduction (ARR), relative risk reduction (RRR) and relative risk (RR) as exact values or point estimates. For example, it may be misleading to say simply that 'warfarin reduces the risk of stroke in patients with atrial fibrillation by 79% (RRR)'. Such an estimate does not accurately reflect uncertainty due to sample size limitations. Thus, in addition to simplistic point estimates, researchers also report an interval estimate which provides a range of possible values of the treatment effect. By convention, interval estimates are estimated at a 95% level of confidence. Thus, when we state 95% confidence intervals (95% CI), we mean that we are 95% sure that the true effect of the treatment lies within this range. Therefore, for warfarin, a better statement would be that 'it reduces the risk of stroke in patients with atrial fibrillation by 79% (RRR), but the actual RRR could range anywhere from 52% to 90%'[5]. By convention, this is expressed as:

$$RRR = 79\% \ [95\% \ CI : 52\%, \ 90\%]$$

How do we interpret the results? Tackle Box 2.3 below summarizes different conclusions that can arise from looking at confidence intervals. Spend some time familiarizing yourself with reading CIs. To make things easier, remember the following four basic tenets.

1. When both ends of the CI are on the side of benefit, the treatment is definitely beneficial.

2. When both ends of the CI are on the side of harm, the treatment is definitely harmful.

3. When one end reflects important benefit and the other end reflects important harm, then the study is inconclusive.

4. When one end reflects a small unimportant benefit and the other end reflects a small unimportant harm, then for all intents and purposes the two treatments being compared are equal.

Confused? Then, you really need to spend time on Tackle Box 2.3. This will be worthwhile as it will help analyse study results quickly and efficiently.

Tackle Box 2.3 demonstrates why it is important to understand confidence intervals. Without them, it would be very difficult to interpret the results of a study. In cases where the 95% CIs are not reported in the article, do not panic! You could either

1. use freely downloadable programs[6,7];

2. call a statistician friend to compute it for you; or

3. compute it yourself[8] (not recommended if you are not confident about working with numbers).

As a final option: go ahead and panic.

2.4 Assessing applicability

After evaluating validity and analysing the results of a trial, the next step is to decide if the results can be applied to our own patients. Trials provide information that can help us decide this. For example, we can check if our patients' characteristics satisfy the inclusion and exclusion criteria. We can also look at treatment effects in subgroups of patients that more closely approximate the individual patient we are trying to help (subgroup analysis). Unfortunately, in real life there are simply too many patient subtypes and trials are typically too small to address more than a few subgroup hypotheses. It would be very unlikely for example, that we find a trial on a drug for hypertension which analyses effects among male smokers aged 40–45, weighing 60–70 kg, with a total cholesterol of 6–7 mmol/Li and a family history of stroke!

Because data from subgroups are limited, healthcare providers must decide on the applicability of trial results to individual patients, based on the general information available to them. In doing this, we suggest consideration of biologic as well as socioeconomic issues.

Biologic issues affecting applicability

Sex

Consider physiological, hormonal or biochemical differences between sexes that might affect the effectiveness of an intervention. For example, women have greater reduction in stroke incidence compared to men when treated with aspirin[9].

Tackle Box 2.3   Interpreting 95% Confidence Intervals (CIs)

Instructions: When researchers express the effect of treatment using the relative risk reduction, absolute risk reduction, or relative risk, they often give us a range of possibilities rather than a single estimate. This range of possibilities is called a '95% Confidence Interval (95% CI)' to mean 'we are 95% sure that the true effect of a drug lies in this range'. Go through this tackle box in rows, to discover how helpful 95% CIs are.

Measure of effectiveness	Interpretation of point estimates	Interpretation of 95% CIs			
		Treatment surely better than control	Treatment surely worse than control	Inconclusive (we need more studies)	The two are probably equivalent
Relative Risk Reduction $$RRR = \frac{R_c - R_t}{R_c}$$	Usually in percent >0% Treatment beneficial ~0% Treatment no effect <0% Treatment harmful	Both ends of 95% CI >0%	Both ends of 95% CI <0%	95% CI straddles 0%; either end is far from 0%	95% CI straddles 0%; either end very close to 0%
		Example: RRR = 7% [95% CI: 6%, 8%]	Example: RRR = −8% [95% CI: −7%, −9%]	Example: RRR = 1% [95% CI: −16%, 15%]	Example: RRR = 0.4% [95% CI: −0.6%, 1.0%]
Absolute Risk Reduction $$ARR = R_c - R_t$$	Usually in percent >0% Treatment beneficial ~0% Treatment no effect <0% Treatment harmful	Both ends of 95% CI > 0%	Both ends of 95% CI < 0%	95% CI wide; straddles 0%	95% CI narrow; straddles 0%
		Example: ARR = 2% [95% CI: 1%, 3%]	Example: ARR = −3% [95% CI: −7%, −1%]	Example: ARR = 1% [95% CI: −9%, 9%]	Example: ARR = 0.2% [95% CI: −0.1%, 0.5%]

Relative Risk $RR = \dfrac{R_t}{R_c}$	Usually in decimals <1.0 Treatment beneficial ~1.0 Treatment no effect >1.0 Treatment harmful	Both ends of 95% CI < 1.0	Both ends of 95% CI > 1.0	95% CI wide; straddles 1.0	95% CI narrow; straddles 1.0
		Example: RR = 0.7 [95% CI: 0.6, 0.8]	Example: RR = 2.4 [95% CI: 1.8, 3.2]	Example: RR = 1 [95% CI: 0.2, 5.3]	Example: RR = 1 [95% CI: 0.9, 1.1]

Note: These interpretations only hold if the dichotomous events are expressed as *adverse* rather than desirable events, e.g. death rather than survival, treatment failure rather that cure, or disease rather than disease-free. When dichotomous outcomes are expressed as desirable events, the interpretation of benefit and harm is reversed. We feel researchers should standardize reporting and use adverse events in order to avoid confusion. Unfortunately, not everyone agrees.

Exercise: An RCT compared stroke rates among patients given an experimental drug or placebo. How would you interpret the following hypothetical results?

(a) RR = 2.3 [95% CI: 1.5, 3.1];
(b) RR = 0.98 [95% CI: 0.95, 1.02];
(c) RR = 0.63 [95% CI: 0.53, 0.73]; and
(d) RR = 0.98 [95% CI: 0.50, 1.50]

Answers: (a) treatment surely worse; (b) the two are equivalent; (c) treatment surely better; and (d) inconclusive results.

Co-Morbidities

Consider co-existent conditions that could affect applicability. Studies show that response to measles vaccination is reduced in malnourished children[10, 11].

Race

Racial differences may affect applicability. For example, black hypertensives are more responsive to diuretics than whites[12]. East Asians are more likely to develop the adverse effect of cough from angiotensin converting enzyme inhibitors compared to whites[13].

Age

Age differences commonly affect response to a treatment. For example, flu vaccines lead to smaller reductions in the risk of influenza in older people[14].

Pathology

Consider differences in the disease under study itself. At times, diseases we refer to by the same name are actually conditions with slightly different pathology. This can lead to significant variations in response to treatment. For example, malaria in Zimbabwe is different from malaria in the Philippines and this is manifested as differences in treatment response[15, 16].

Socioeconomic issues affecting applicability

Most trials are carried out under ideal conditions, which are difficult to apply in everyday life. This is as much a problem of provider compliance as it is a problem of patient compliance. Patient compliance problems often relate to markers of socioeconomic disadvantage such as poverty and lack of education. Provider compliance problems, on the other hand, are often related to skill in the implementation of certain procedures and availability of necessary facilities. Some therapies present both types of compliance problems. Warfarin administration for atrial fibrillation, for example, requires not only strict patient compliance with monitoring, but also availability of resources for prothrombin time determination and emergency management of life-threatening bleeds.

2.5 Individualizing the results

When you are satisfied that biologic and socioeconomic factors will not compromise effectiveness, the next step is to individualize the benefit, risks and costs to your patient. While studies report effectiveness of a treatment in a population as a whole, the benefits, risks and costs will vary slightly from patient to patient. The main source of this variation is the patient's baseline risk for the event you are trying to prevent. Variation in risk is very common in medicine. Patients have mild, moderate or severe forms of the same disease, or may have variable risk factors for an adverse outcome. Some individuals may come in early and others may come in late in the course of an illness. Tackle Box 2.4 shows us five quick steps in using the baseline risk to estimate the effect of therapy on an individual.

You now have information on the individualized benefits, harms and costs of treatment which you can use to reach a decision for your patient. Remember that we tend to make decisions for patients most of the time. This is acceptable for treatments where benefits far outweigh the harm, and cost is not a problem. However, when we are at a deadlock between benefit and harm, or when cost is potentially prohibitive, we may want to provide information for our patient in a clear and concise but

Tackle Box 2.4 Steps to estimate the individualized changes in risk

Instructions: Studies estimate the average effect of treatment on groups of people, but unfortunately, not everyone is average. Some people have milder disease than average, while others have more severe disease. Consideration of these differences allows us to individualize the estimated effect of treatment. Here are five simple steps to do this.

Step	How to do it	Example: Treatment showing benefit	Example: Treatment showing harm
Step 1: Estimate your individual patient's risk for an event *without* treatment (R_c).	This is estimated from clinical features of the patient's condition, e.g. severity, stage of disease, age, risk factors, etc. Possible references include studies on prognosis. For a few diseases, risk calculators are available (e.g. coronary risk calculators).[17,18]	A 55-year old male with atrial fibrillation, diabetes hypertension, a prior stroke but no valve disease has an annual risk of ischemic stroke of 8%[19].	A 55-year old male with atrial fibrillation, diabetes hypertension, a prior stroke but no valve disease has a small annual risk of major extracranial haemorrhage of approximately 1%[20].
Step 2: Estimate the RR using the study results.	If the relative risk (RR) is given, well and good. If not, estimate it from the relative risk reduction (RRR). Simply convert RRR from percent to decimal notation and subtract from 1.00. For example, if RRR = 25%, then RR = 1.00 − 0. 25 = 0.75.	If we give warfarin to the patient above, we can reduce the risk of an ischemic stroke: RR = 0.36[19]	If we give warfarin to the patient above, we increase the risk of a extracranial haemorrhage: RR = 4.3[19]

Step 3: Estimate your individual patient's risk for an event *with* treatment (R_t).	$RR = \dfrac{R_t}{R_c}$, therefore $R_t = R_c \times RR$	$R_t = R_c \times RR$ $= 8\% \times 0.36$ $= 2.9\%$	$R_t = R_c \times RR$ $= 1\% \times 4.3$ $= 4.3\%$
Step 4: Estimate the individualized absolute risk reduction (ARR)	$ARR = R_c - R_t$ (from step 1 and 3)	$ARR = 8.0\% - 2.9\%$ $= 5.1\%$	ARR $= 1\% - 4.3\%$ $= -3.3\%$
Step 5: Estimate the individualized number needed to treat (NNT) or number needed to harm (NNH)	$NNT = 100/ARR$	$NNT = 100/5.1 = 20$	$NNT = 100/-3.3 = -30$ or $NNH = 30$

Note: Sometimes your only source for step 1 is the control group in the trials themselves. If this is the case, then you don't need to go through all five steps. The individualized NNT for your patient is the one reported in the study.

Exercises:

1. What would the NNT be in the example in column 3, if the baseline risk for ischemic stroke was (a) 16%; (b) 32%?
2. What would the NNH be in the example in column 4, if the baseline risk for extracranial haemorrhage was (a) 2%; (b) 4%?

Answers: 1(a) 10; 1(b) 5; 2(a) 15; 2(b) 7

balanced manner. Tools that have been used for this purpose are called *patient decision aids*. They may take the form of audio or video tapes, illustrations or reading materials, and have been shown to improve knowledge as well as stimulate participation in decision-making[21].

Patients are unlikely to understand RR, RRR or ARR easily, so a better way to express treatment effects would be to simply show them the changes in risk. Using the example of warfarin for patients with atrial fibrillation but no valve disease (Tackle Box 2.4), we might summarize the individualized effect of treatment as follows.

> Benefit: The risk of ischemic stroke falls from 8.0% to 2.9% per year.
> Harm: The risk of haemorrhagic stroke rises from 1.0% to 4.3% per year.
> Cost: Average treatment cost would be US $365 per year (based on Philippine prices as of 2007).

Unfortunately, presenting information in this way may be challenging for many patients[22]. An effective way of simplifying this would be to present a face table[23, 24]. Face tables consist of 100 faces, coloured or shaded to indicate the probability of certain outcomes. In the example in Figure 2.2, two sets of 100 faces represent treated and untreated patients. White 'smiley' faces

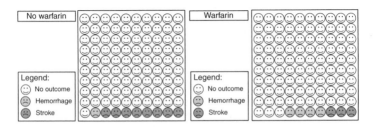

Figure 2.2 Face table summarizing the effect of warfarin in a patient with atrial fibrillation but no valve disease

represent patients who do well, dark grey 'frowny' faces represent patients who develop the unfavourable outcome being prevented (e.g. stroke), and the light grey 'frowny' faces represent the number with an adverse effect (e.g. extracranial haemorrhage). Decision aids such as these face tables enable patients to visualize the trade-offs between benefit and harm better than numbers can.

2.6 Summary

Articles on therapy are probably the most common types of articles that we come across. When confronted with a therapy article, first appraise directness: does it directly address a question that is important to you? If it does, appraise validity to decide if the results are credible. Try to save yourself some time. You don't need to read the entire article. Just go straight ahead and seek answers to each of the validity questions. If you are satisfied that the study is valid, proceed to appraise the results. However, do not simply accept the findings hook-line-and-sinker. Remember, you still have to assess applicability. If you are satisfied with directness, validity, the results and applicability, then individualize the results to estimate specific effects on your individual patient. Involve them in decisions when necessary, by sharing what you know about risks, benefits and costs.

References

[1] Grady D, Chaput L and Kristof M. 2003. Results of Systematic Review of Research on Diagnosis and Treatment of Coronary Heart Disease in Women, Evidence Report/Technology Assessment No. 80. University of California, San Francisco-Stanford Evidence-Based Practice Center. AHRQ Publication No. 03-E035.
[2] Chobanian AV, Bakris GL, Black HR, Cushman WC, Green LA, Izzo JL Jr, Jones DW, Materson BJ, Oparil S, Wright JT Jr and

Roccella EJ. 2003. Joint National Committee on Prevention, Detection, Evaluation, and Treatment of High Blood Pressure. National Heart, Lung, and Blood Institute; National High Blood Pressure Education Program Coordinating Committee. Seventh report of the Joint National Committee on Prevention, Detection, Evaluation, and Treatment of High Blood Pressure. *Hypertension.* 42(6): 1206–1252. Epub 2003 Dec 1. http://www.nhlbi.nih.gov/guidelines/hypertension/express.pdf

[3] Epstein AE, Bigger JT, Wyse DG, Romhilt DW, Reynolds-Haertle RA and Hallstrom AP. 1991. Events in the Cardiac Arrhythmia Suppression Trial (CAST): mortality in the entire population enrolled. *Journal of American College of Cardiology.* 18(1): 14–19.

[4] Moore TJ. 1995. *Deadly Medicine.* Simon & Schuster: New York.

[5] Ezekowitz MD, Bridgers SL, James KE, Carliner NH, Colling CL and Gornick CC. 1992. Warfarin in the prevention of stroke associated with nonrheumatic atrial fibrillation. Veterans affairs stroke prevention in nonrheumatic atrial fibrillation investigators. *New England Journal of Medicine.* 327: 1406–1412.

[6] http://www.cdc.gov/epiinfo/epiinfo.htm

[7] http://www.statpac.com/statistics-calculator/index.htm

[8] Riffenburgh RH. 2006. *Statistics in Medicine.* Second Edition. Academic Press: USA.

[9] Ridker PM, Cook NR, Lee I, Gordon D, Gaziano JM, Manson JE, Hennekens CH and Buring JE. 2005. A randomized trial of low-dose aspirin in the primary prevention of cardiovascular disease in women. *New England Journal of Medicine.* 13(352): 1293–1304.

[10] Adu FD, Akinwolere OA, Tomori O and Uche LN. 1992. Low seroconversion rates to measles vaccine among children in Nigeria. *Bulletin of World Health Organisation.* 70: 457–460.

[11] Bautista-Lopez N, Vaisberg A, Kanashiro R, Hernandez H and Ward BJ. 2001. Immune response to measles vaccine in Peruvian children. *Bulletin of World Health Organisation.* 79: 1038–1046.

[12] Falkner B and Kushner H. 1990. Effect of chronic sodium loading on cardiovascular response in young blacks and whites. *Hypertension.* 15: 36–43.

[13] McDowell SE, Coleman JJ and Ferner RE. 2006. Systematic review and meta-analysis of ethnic differences in risks of adverse reactions to drugs used in cardiovascular medicine. *British Medical Journal.* 332: 1177–1181. DOI 10.1136/bmj.38803.528113.55.

[14] Villari P, Manzoli L and Boccia A. 2004. Methodological quality of studies and patient age as major sources of variation in efficacy esti-

mates of influenza vaccination in healthy adults: a meta-analysis. *Vaccine.* **22**(25–26): 3475–3486.

[15] Mharakurwa S, Manyame B and Shiff CJ. 1997. Trial of the ParaSight-F test for malaria diagnosis in the primary health care system, Zimbabwe. *Tropical Medicine/International Health.* **2**: 544–550.

[16] Bell D, Go R, Miguel C, Walker J, Cacal L and Saul A. 2001. Diagnosis of malaria in a remote area of the Philippines: comparison of techniques and their acceptance by health workers and the community. *Bulletin of World Health Organisation.* **79**: 933–941.

[17] http://www.intmed.mcw.edu/clincalc/heartrisk.html

[18] http://www.chd-taskforce.com/calculator/calculator.htm

[19] Rothman KJ. 2002. *Epidemiology.* Chapter 3. Oxford University Press: Oxford; p. 46–49.

[20] Saxena R and Koudstaal PJ. 2004. Anticoagulants for preventing stroke in patients with nonrheumatic atrial fibrillation and a history of stroke or transient ischaemic attack. *Cochrane Database of Systematic Reviews.* **2**:CD000185. DOI: 10.1002/14651858.CD000185.pub2.

[21] O'Connor AM, Stacey D, Rovner D, Holmes-Rovner M, Tetroe J, Llewellyn-Thomas H, Entwistle V, Rostom A, Fiset V, Barry M and Jones J. 2001. Decision aids for people facing health treatment or screening decisions. *Cochrane Database of Systematic Reviews.* **3**:CD001431. Update in 2003 **2**:CD001431.

[22] Edwards A, Hood K, Matthews EJ, Russell D, Russell IT, Barker J, Pill R and Stott N. 2000. The effectiveness of one-to-one risk communication interventions in health care: a systematic review. *Medical Decision Making.* **20**: 290–297.

[23] Santesso N, Maxwell L, Tugwell PS, Wells GA, O'Connor AM, Judd M and Buchbinder R. 2006. Knowledge transfer to clinicians and consumers by the Cochrane Musculoskeletal Group. *Journal of Rheumatology.* **33**(11): 2312–2318.

[24] Feldman-Stewart D, Kocovski N, McConnell BA, Brundage MD, and Mackillop WJ. 2000. Perception of quantitative information for treatment decisions. *Medical Decision Making.* **20**: 228.

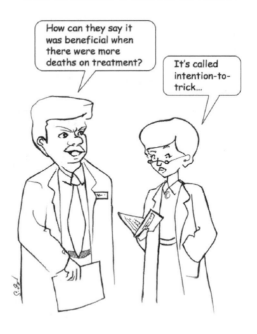

3

Evaluation of Articles on Diagnosis

Maria Asuncion A. Silvestre, Aldrin B. Loyola, Antonio L. Dans, Leonila F. Dans

Tests may be performed for various reasons, including to

1. plan an intervention (e.g. surgery);

2. monitor response to therapy;

3. estimate risk of future events; or

4. determine prognosis in patients with a known disease.

This chapter deals with studies that evaluate a fifth function of tests, which is to diagnose the presence or absence of a particular condition.

Painless Evidence-Based Medicine   Antonio L. Dans, Leonila F. Dans and Maria Asuncion A. Silvestre
© 2008 John Wiley & Sons, Ltd

3.1 Appraising directness

Questions on diagnosis should be phrased in terms of the following variables: P, the patient population on whom the test might be done; E, the exposure (in this case the test to be performed); and O, the outcome (i.e. the condition that the test is supposed to diagnose). Examples include:

> Among postmenopausal women presenting with a breast mass (P), how accurate is fine needle aspiration biopsy (E) in establishing the presence or absence of breast cancer (O)?

> In Bacille Calmette Guerin (BCG)-vaccinated children (P), how accurate is an interferon-γ assay (E) in establishing the presence or absence of tuberculosis (O)?

As in articles on therapy, before even reading an article, the first thing we must do is evaluate directness i.e. how well the PEO in the study (the research question), corresponds with your own PEO (the clinical question). Did the study evaluate the kind of patients you are interested in? Is the test in the study exactly the one you want? Is the disease which is being diagnosed the same? If you feel the article might provide a reasonably close answer to the question you ask, then proceed to evaluate it in greater detail. Otherwise, it would be wiser to spend your time on something else.

3.2 Appraising validity

Question #1: Was the reference standard an acceptable one?

To measure the accuracy of a particular test we need to compare its results to a *reference standard*, a test that can unequivocally establish presence or absence of the disease in question. Unfortunately, perfect tests are very rare and when they do exist, they tend to be invasive and expensive. Because of this, researchers evaluating diagnostic tests spend a lot of time trying to strike a balance between cost, accuracy and safety in choosing a reference standard.

While many single tests (such as histopathologic examinations) are considered classic examples of reference standards, such tests do not always work for complex conditions. Sometimes, researchers resort to establishing disease presence using multiple criteria (e.g. the Jones criteria to diagnose rheumatic fever)[1] or even response to therapy (e.g. reversible airway obstruction to diagnose bronchial asthma)[2]. Whatever they choose, they must ensure that their reference standard defines disease in a way that is *acceptable* to medical practitioners.

Conceptualizing reference standards as *acceptable* rather than *exact* definitions of disease makes the lives of researchers easier. It means they can choose a reference standard on the basis of feasibility, even if it is not the most accurate of several choices. While this may seem unscientific, it approximates what actually happens in real life. In real life, a simple sputum AFB stain is used more often than an expensive AFB culture for the diagnosis of pulmonary tuberculosis[3]. Similarly, in the diagnosis of minimal change disease (MCD), the response to a therapeutic trial of steroids is an acceptable alternative to a kidney biopsy[4–6]. The point is if clinicians are willing to make treatment decisions based on these definitions of disease, then surely researchers can use these definitions as reference standards. A common approach is to use disease definitions officially adopted by specialty organizations. These can usually be found in consensus statements that they publish (e.g. the definition of antiphospholipid antibody syndrome in pregnancy)[7].

Question #2: Was the reference standard interpreted independently from the test in question?

Since the accuracy of the test in question is gauged by how often its results agree with the results of the reference standard, measures should be taken to ensure that knowledge of the results of one test does not bias interpretation of the other. This is not as easy as it sounds. Many studies on diagnosis are performed retrospectively using data already collected for clinical reasons. Medical records, for example, are commonly used. Although the retrospective nature of such studies makes them more feasible, assurance of independent interpretation becomes much more difficult for several reasons.

1. In most situations, there is no perceived need to maintain independence. In fact, it is standard practice when requesting some tests to supply the laboratory with information on prior findings. For example, clinical data is routinely supplied to the interpreter, prior to performance of a chest x-ray.

2. The result of a test often becomes the indication for performing the reference standard. This allows one test to influence performance and interpretation of the other. For example, if the result of a needle aspiration biopsy of a breast mass is positive, it is more likely that the individual will be subjected to an excision biopsy.

3. Other times, the result of the test itself is part of the reference standard (e.g. the results of a tuberculin skin test such as the PPD test is often part of multi-criteria definition of tuberculosis)[8]. As such, the test and reference standard are not strictly independent.

Not only are these three pitfalls difficult to avoid for authors, they are difficult for us to spot as readers. Authors will simply say that both the test and the reference standard were performed in all patients. They will rarely point out that, at least in some of the cases they analysed, the interpretation of the tests was not independent. Perhaps the biggest clue that this may have happened is when the study is conducted in a retrospective manner e.g. chart reviews.

3.3 Appraising results

Question # 1: What were the likelihood ratios of the various test results?

After performing the two tests (the test being evaluated against the reference standard) on the study patients, the conventional method of comparing results in a 2×2 table is shown in Tackle Box 3.1. Consider this table for a few minutes before proceeding. If you already understand the concepts of sensitivity, specificity and predictive values, you may want to skip this table altogether.

The main problem with sensitivity, specificity and predictive values is that they only work in situations where the test being evaluated has two results. In truth, tests with just two results (positive or negative) are unusual. They only seem common for the following two reasons.

1. Researchers like to set cutoffs when tests have many results e.g. a home pregnancy test is actually a measurement of urinary HCG titers; it only seems to have two results because the colour change of the test strip is set to occur at a certain level[9].

2. Researchers like to ignore the meaning of intermediate results e.g. fine needle aspiration biopsy of breast nodules was reported as definitely malignant or definitely benign in one study, but there were actually equivocal results which were ignored in the analysis[10].

Tackle Box 3.1   Comparing the results of a test with a reference standard when the test has only two results, e.g. positive or negative

Instructions: Standard symbols are used in the 2×2 table below: $a =$ the number of persons with a *true positive* result (test is positive and person has disease); $b =$ the number of persons with a *false positive* result (test is positive and person has no disease); $c =$ the number of persons with a *false negative* result (test is negative and person has disease); $d =$ the number of persons with a *true negative* result (test is negative and person has no disease); $(a + c) =$ number of persons with the disease; $(b + d) =$ number of persons without the disease; $(a + b) =$ number of persons with a positive test; $(c + d) =$ number of persons with a negative test. Go through the formulae below to discover different ways of reporting concordance between the test and the gold standard.

Test result	Reference standard		
	Disease present	Disease absent	Row total
Positive	a	b	(a + b)
Negative	c	d	(c + d)
Column total	(a + c)	(b + d)	

Notes: Using the variables a, b, c and d, there are four traditional ways of expressing how correct a test is.

1. *Sensitivity* (sn) refers to the proportion of persons with disease who correctly have a positive test, i.e. $a/(a + c)$;
2. *Specificity* (sp) refers to the proportion of persons with no disease who correctly have a negative test, i.e. $d/(b + d)$.
3. *Positive predictive value* (ppv) is the proportion of persons with a positive test who correctly turn out to have disease, i.e. $a/(a + b)$;
4. *Negative predictive value* (npv) is the proportion of persons with a negative test who correctly turn out to have no disease, i.e. $d/(c + d)$.

These numbers are not difficult to remember. The denominators for sn and sp are the column totals, i.e. they are the proportions of correct results in *columns* 1 and 2 respectively. The denominators for ppv and npv are the row totals, i.e. they are the proportions of correct results in *rows* 1 and 2, respectively.

Exercise: Assume $a = 42$, $b = 7$, $c = 4$ and $d = 38$. Compute (a) sn, (b) sp, (c) ppv and (d) npv

Answers: (a) 91.3%, (b) 84.4%, (c) 85.7% and (d) 90.5%

To evaluate a test with multi-level results, a 2×2 table will not suffice. We need a '$2 \times n$' table where n is the number of results that a test may have. Instead of sensitivity, specificity and predictive values, we will need a relatively new measure of accuracy: the likelihood ratio (LR). Study Tackle Box 3.2 for a few minutes before proceeding, to understand likelihood ratios. It is not important to comprehend the formulae for calculating LR, as long as it is understood that LR is a measure of how much the likelihood of disease changes given a test result.

3.4   Assessing applicability

If you think the study is reasonably valid and that the results show acceptable accuracy, the next step is to evaluate applicability to your particular patient. As in evaluating articles on therapy, biologic and socioeconomic issues may affect how well the test performs in the real world.

Biologic issues affecting applicability

Sex

Consider physiological, hormonal or biochemical differences between males and females that might affect the test results. For example, creatinine clearance based on a single serum creatinine determination must be adjusted according to sex[11].

Co-morbidities

Consider co-morbid conditions that could affect the performance of the diagnostic examination. For example, malnutrition can decrease sensitivity of a tuberculin skin test[12].

Tackle Box 3.2   Comparing the results of a test with a reference standard when the test has two or more results, e.g. positive, intermediate or negative

Instructions: Standard symbols are used in the 2 × n table below: a = the number of persons with disease and a positive result; b = the number of persons without disease but a positive result; c = number of persons with disease and an intermediate result; d = number of persons without disease and an intermediate result; e = number of persons with disease but a negative result; f = number of persons without disease and a negative result. There may be more cells depending on how many intermediate results there are. Go through the formulae below to discover different ways of reporting concordance between the test and the gold standard.

Test result	Reference standard		
	Disease present	Disease absent	Row total
Positive	a	b	(a + b)
Intermediate	c	d	(c + d)
Negative	e	f	(e + f)
Column Total	(a + c + e)	(b + d + f)	

Notes:

1) At this point, it is important to distinguish between probabilities and odds. Probabilities are portions of the whole, while odds are the ratio of portions. Say that again? Well, if we were talking of a pie (figure in right), probability would be a piece of the pie divided by the entire pie, i.e. a/(a + b). Odds, on
the other hand, would be a piece of the pie divided by the rest of the pie, i.e. a/b. To convert from probability to odds, we simply reduce the denominator by subtracting the numerator from it. For example: 7/100 (probability) becomes 7/93 (odds); 92/100 (probability) becomes 92/8 (odds).

2) The odds of disease when the test is positive is the ratio of a to b. This is written as a:b or a/b. It is read as 'a is to b'. Similarly, the odds of disease when the test is intermediate are c/d. When the test is negative, the odds are e/f. There may be g/h, i/j and so forth depending on the number of intermediate results. The overall odds of disease regardless of the test results is (a + c + e)/(b + d + f). This is also the odds of disease regardless of test results, most commonly referred to as the **pre-test odds**.

3) These odds may be used to estimate likelihood ratios (LRs) for each result. The LR is nothing more than the odds of disease given a test result (the **post-test odds**), divided by the overall odds of disease (the **pre-test odds**).

Thus for a positive test, the LR is $(a/b) \div [(a+c+e)/(b+d+f)]$. For an intermediate test, the LR is $(c/d) \div [(a+c+e)/(b+d+f)]$. Finally, for a negative test, the LR is $(e/f) \div [(a+c+e)/(b+d+f)]$. (If you cannot perform any of the above operations because the denominator is 0, impute a value of 1 for that cell and adjust the corresponding column or row total.)

4) If the LRs are not provided, you may need to compute your own by reconstructing a $2 \times n$ table from the data provided. If sensitivity and specificity are reported, reconstruct the $2 \times n$ table by assigning a = sensitivity, b = 100 – specificity, c = 100 – sensitivity, and d = specificity. Then compute for LR as described in step 3.

5) Because LR is the ratio of post-test to pre-test odds, it is an expression of change in the odds of disease. Thus an LR of 10/1 represents a 10-fold increase in the odds of disease, while an LR of 1/10 (or 0.1) expresses a 10-fold drop in the odds of disease. Similarly, an LR of 1/1 (or 1.0) represents a test result that does not change the odds of disease. Thus, the further away from 1.0 the LR is, the greater the rise or fall in odds of disease.

Exercise:

1. Assume a = 35, b = 10, c = 10, d = 20, e = 5 and f = 70. Calculate
   (a) LR of a positive test result, (b) LR of intermediate test results and
   (c) LR of a negative test result.
2. If sn = 90 and sp = 60, what would be the LR of a (a) positive test and a
   (b) negative test? Clue: reconstruct the $2 \times n$ table as advised in note #4 above.

Answers: 1(a) 7.00, 1(b) 1.00, 1(c) 0.14, 2(a) 2.25, 2(b) 0.17

Race

Consider racial differences that may alter the performance of the test in question. For example, African-American ancestry increased the likelihood of high grade prostate cancer in patients with high levels of prostate specific antigen[13].

Age

Consider the age of the population in the study in relation to your own patients. A sputum AFB stain performs well in adults but gastric aspirates would maximize accuracy in infants[14].

Pathology

Test accuracy is influenced by the severity and duration of the patient's illness. In general, the more advanced a disease is, the easier it is to diagnose. For this reason, studies on hospitalized patients (i.e. patients with severe disease) can sometimes lead to overestimates of the accuracy of a test. Knowing where a trial was done gives you an idea of the kinds of patients recruited, and can help you decide whether you can still use the authors' conclusions.

Socioeconomic issues affecting applicability

The accuracy of questionnaires is particularly prone to social, cultural and economic differences among patients. One reason is that a lot can be lost in the translation of questionnaires. However, even if the language used is the same, interpretation and reaction may vary. For example, cognitive tests tend to underestimate the abilities of elderly people from ethnic minorities. This can lead to overdiagnosis of dementia in these communities[15]. The CAGE questionnaire (which is commonly used to detect alcoholism) performed poorly in some ethnic groups, particularly African-American men[16]. Similarly, a questionnaire to detect autism developed in the US and UK could not be used in families in Hong Kong because of perceived cultural differences[17]. These examples (and many more) should lead us to look for local validation studies before accepting the accuracy of diagnostic tests, especially in the form of questionnaires.

Even laboratory tests may sometimes have questionable applicability. When your laboratory has limited resources, it may not match the standards of performance defined in a study which uses the best equipment, hires the best diagnosticians and continuously monitors good laboratory practice. We need to ensure that these standards are (at least) approximated by the local laboratories we use.

3.5   Individualizing the results

When satisfied that biologic and socioeconomic differences do not compromise the applicability of a test in your setting, the next step is to determine the impact that the test (and its results) might have on your specific patient's probability of having a disease. While studies of diagnosis report the average effect of a test on probability of disease, the effect may vary greatly from patient to patient. The main source of this variation is the individual's baseline probability of disease, also known as the pre-test probability.

A variation in pre-test probability is common. Based on history and physical examination, individuals may have little or no signs of disease in which case disease probability is very low. Other individuals may have florid signs of disease, in which case the pre-test probability is very high. Take, for example, a 24-year old female consulting for fleeting chest pain. Her history reveals occasional pricking pain on the anterior chest wall not related to effort. Her physical findings are unremarkable. The probability that this particular individual is having a heart attack is quite low, i.e. you assess her pre-test probability for a heart attack to be around 0.1%. Contrast this with a 60-year hypertensive male smoker with a chronic history of chest discomfort during physical exertion. He presents at the emergency room with acute, severe chest pain. On physical examination, he is hypotensive with a BP of 80/60, tachycardic with a heart rate of 110 and has cold clammy perspiration. The probability of this man having a heart attack is high, i.e. the pre-test probability of a heart attack may

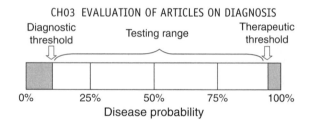

Figure 3.1 Disease probability and thresholds of management

be more than 90%. Figure 3.1 above illustrates the probability of disease, and shows us some conceptual thresholds in the management of disease.

Figure 3.1 depicts the two threshold regions at the upper and lower levels of probability: the therapeutic threshold is the probability of disease above which we are willing to stop testing and just get on with therapy and the diagnostic threshold is the probability of disease below which we are willing to stop testing and just reassure the patient. Between these two thresholds, the clinician is more uncertain and so further tests are required. Tests are useful when they can move us out of the testing range to somewhere beyond the treatment threshold (so we can commence treatment), or below the diagnostic threshold (so we can just reassure the patient or consider other diseases). How do the results of a test change disease probability i.e. how do we estimate the *post-test probability*? Tackle Box 3.3 illustrates a strategy for those who are up to the challenge of manual computation. Tackle Box 3.4 illustrates a strategy for those of us afraid of numbers.

After arriving at a post-test probability of disease, you may now make a clinical decision, i.e. to treat, reassure, or carry out more tests (depending on whether you land above the treatment threshold, below the diagnostic threshold or in-between).

While this discussion focuses on use of likelihood ratios to interpret test results when they arrive, we can also use these calculations to decide if the tests should be done at all for a particular patient. Consider the following when you contemplate requesting a test.

1. When the test result will not lead to important changes in probability, we should think twice about doing the test at all. Remember that the change in probability is not just a function of the LRs of a test, it is also a function of the pre-test probability. When the pre-test probability is close to 50% (as uncertain as it can get), the changes in probability tend to be great and the tests become much more useful. When the pre-test probability is already close to 0% or 100%, the changes in probability tend to be very small and testing is of less value.

2. When effective treatment is unavailable for the disease you are detecting, either because it is difficult to treat or the patient cannot afford the treatment, testing may not be useful.

3. The cost of the test should always be considered, especially in places where medical care is mainly an out-of-pocket expense. When we talk of cost, it is not just the immediate cost of the test but also the cost of the subsequent tests, as well as subsequent medical or surgical interventions.

4. Safety is an issue for some tests, especially invasive procedures.

5. Just as we should involve the patient when deciding on a therapeutic intervention, the patient should make informed choices about diagnostic tests to be performed.

Tackle Box 3.3 Computing for post-test probability of disease given a test result

Instructions: Results of a test change the probability of disease. This tackle box discusses the math involved. If you're numero-phobic, skip this tackle box and proceed directly to Tackle Box 3.4.

	How to do this	Need an equation?
Step 1: Estimate the pre-test probability in percent.	Interview the patient and carry out a good physical examination. Based on your findings, your clinical experience will give you a good estimate of the probability of disease. If the case is difficult, an expert might be in a better position to estimate what the probability of the disease might be. Exercise (1): Ms X, a 25-year old sexually active female presents with a 3-day history of burning sensation on urination. Physical exam was unremarkable. Estimate the pre-test probability that she has a urinary tract infection (UTI).	There isn't any . . . what you need are good skills in history and physical examination.
Step 2: Convert pre-test probability to odds.	There are two ways of expressing the possibility of disease: as odds or as probabilities. Probabilities are a portion of the whole, while odds are the ratio of portions. To convert from probability to odds, we simply reduce the denominator by subtracting the numerator from it. For example: 25/100 (probability) becomes 25/75 (odds), and 90/100 (probability) becomes 90/10 (odds). If you are not yet comfortable with probabilities and odds, return to Tackle Box 3.2 (review the concept of the pie)! Exercise [2]: If you set the pre-test probability of UTI in exercise [1] at 80%, what would the pre-test odds be?	$$\text{Odds} = \frac{\text{Probability}}{100 - \text{Probability}}$$

Step 3: Multiply pre-test odds by the Likelihood Ratio of the test result to get the post-test odds.	The pre-test odds were estimated in step 2. The study you read should tell you the LR of the test result you obtained. Remember, LR varies according to the result. A positive test will probably have an LR > 1.0, a negative test an LR < 1.0 while an equivocal test an LR that is close to 1.0.	Post-test Odds = Pre-test Odds × LR
	Exercise (3): Continuing the scenario in exercise (2), estimate the post-test odds of UTI in the following scenarios: (a) her urine dipstick nitrite is positive; (b) her urine dipstick is negative. Note: Study shows that urine dipstick nitrite has an LR(+) = 3.0 and an LR(−) = 0.5^{18}.	
Step 4: Convert post-test odds back to post-test probability in percent.	Simple. Just increase the denominator by adding the numerator back to it. Thus, odds of 1/3 become a probability of 1/4 (or 25%); and odds of 1/1 become a probability of 1/2 (or 50%). You can also use the formula in the next column. Exercise (4): Convert the post-test odds back to (post-test) probability in the two scenarios in exercise (3).	$$\text{Probability} = \frac{\text{Odds}}{1+\text{Odds}} \times 100$$

Notes:

1. In these equations, probability is expressed as a percentage.

2. Usually a sequence of tests is necessary to confirm disease or rule it out. In this case, the post-test probability of one test becomes the pre-test probability for the next test and so forth. This only works in non-emergency cases. When confronted with an emergency, forget sequential tests; do everything at the same time!

Answers: Exercise (1): Depending on the details of the history, estimates of the probability of UTI may vary. A reasonable estimate might be around 80%. Exercise (2): If you set the pre-test probability at 80%, pre-test odds will be 80/20 or 4/1. Exercise (3): For scenario (a) with urine dipstick result positive, post-test odds = 4.0 × 3.0 = 12. For scenario (b) with urine dipstick result negative, post-test odds = 4.0 × 0.5 = 2. Exercise (4): For scenario (a), post-test probability will be [12/(1+12)] x 100 = 92%. For scenario (b), post-test probability will be [2/(1 + 2)] × 100 = 67%.

Tackle Box 3.4   Estimating post-test probability of disease given test results (using nomogram [18])

Instructions: If you are uncomfortable with manual computations for post-test probability as described in tackle box 3.3, go through the nomogram shown in Figure 3.2 to learn an easier way to do it.

Step 1: Estimate the pre-test probability based on your history or physical examination, i.e. clinical intuition. You can also derive this estimate from the results of surveys. Plot this on the left-most vertical axis.

Exercise: Ms X, a 25-year old sexually active female presents with a three day history of a burning sensation on urination. Physical exam was unremarkable. Estimate the pre-test probability that she has a urinary tract infection (UTI).

Step 2: Determine the likelihood ratio of the test result from the results of the study you reviewed. Remember, the LR varies depending on the test result. Plot this on the middle vertical axis.

Exercise: Study shows that urine dipstick nitrite has an LR(+) = 3.0 and LR(−) = 0.5[19]. Look for these points along the middle axis.

Step 3: Connect the two points in steps 1 and 2, and extend the line to the rightmost vertical axis. The point of intersection is the probability of disease after the test (the post-test probability).

Exercise: What would the post-test probabilities be if (a) her dipstick nitrite is positive; (b) her dipstick nitrite is negative?

Note: Sometimes, a sequence of tests is necessary to confirm disease or rule it out. In this case, the post-test probability of the earlier test becomes the pre-test probability for the next test and so forth and so on. This only works in non-emergency cases. When confronted with an emergency, forget about sequential testing, do everything at the same time!

Answers: If you set the pre-test probability at 80%, if the urine dipstick result is positive, post-test probability will be around 95% and when negative, the post-test probability will be around 65%. These numbers just approximate the exact answers for Tackle Box 3.3.

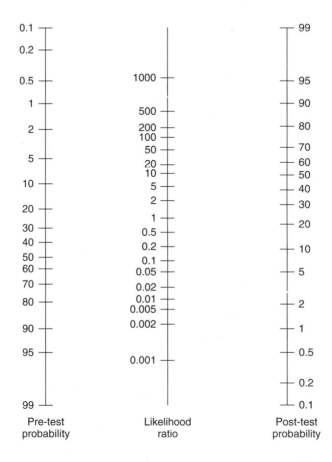

Figure 3.2 Bayes nomogram for estimating post-test probability*
* Reproduced with permission[18]

3.6   Summary

Articles on diagnostic tests are sometimes considered difficult reading. By dissecting them one step at a time, the task becomes simple and straightforward. First appraise directness: is the question asked important to you? Is the test something you are considering? Is it available? Is it a feasible option? If not, maybe you should be looking for another article. If it does address an important question for you, the next step is to appraise validity. This will tell you if the results are credible. If the results aren't credible anyway, why even bother appraising the article? These two steps can save you lots of time spent on futile reading.

If you decide to proceed and interpret the results, look for likelihood ratios, or (heaven forbid) information that may lead you to compute them yourself. Before actually using these numbers, however, decide if the information is applicable to your setting. Biologic and socioeconomic factors should be considered.

If everything is in order (directness, validity, results and applicability), you now have information to:

1. decide if the test is something you would like to request, and

2. interpret the results when they arrive.

Don't become too engrossed with numbers. Sometimes it's enough just to understand that LRs are a measure of changes in disease probability. Test results with LR > 1.0 increase the disease probability. The higher the LR is, the closer it can bring you to confirming the disease. Test results with LR < 1.0 decrease the disease probability. The lower the LR is, the closer it can bring you to ruling out disease. Test results with LR very close to 1.0 have little impact on your clinical or pre-test estimates of disease probability.

When you have arrived at your post-test probability of disease, you can now make a clinical decision based on your thresholds of management and also your patient's preferences. There are usually three choices:

1. stop testing and get on with the treatment of the probable disease;

2. stop testing and reassure the patient that disease probability is low; or

3. do more tests before you decide.

References

[1] Ferrieri P for the Jones Criteria Working Group. 2002. Proceedings of the Jones Criteria Workshop. *Circulation.* **106**: 2521.

[2] Boulet LP, Becker A, Berube D, Beveridge D and Ernst P. 1999. Canadian asthma consensus report, 1999. Canadian Asthma Consensus Group. Diagnosis and evaluation of asthma in adults. *Canadian Medical Association Journal.* **161**(11) S6–S7.

[3] Sennik D. 2006. BMJ Review. Pulmonary tuberculosis: diagnosis and treatment. *BMJ Clinical Review.* **332**: 1194–1197.

[4] Gulati S, Sharma AP, Sharma RK, Gupta A and Gupta RK. 2002. Do current recommendations for kidney biopsy in nephritic syndrome need modifications? *Pediatric Nephrology.* **17**: 404–408.

[5] Gandhi BV. 1994. The role of renal biopsy in nephrotic syndrome. *Journal of Postgraduate Medicine.* **40**: 135–136.

[6] Filler G, Young E, Geier P, Carpenter B, Drukker A and Feber J. 2003. Is there really an increase in non-minimal change nephrotic syndrome in children? *American Journal of Kidney Diseases.* **42**(6): 1107–1113.

[7] Wilson WA, Gharavi AE, Koike T, Lockshin MD, Branch DW, Piette JC, Brey R, Derksen R, Harris EN, Hughes GR, Triplett DA and Khamashta MA. 1999. International consensus statement on preliminary classification criteria for definite APS: report of an international workshop. *Arthritis & Rheumatism.* **42**: 1309–1311.

[8] Taylor Z, Nolan CM and Blumberg HM. 2005. American Thoracic Society; Centers for Disease Control and Prevention; Infectious

Diseases Society of America. Controlling tuberculosis in the United States. Recommendations from the American Thoracic Society, CDC, and the Infectious Diseases Society of America. *Morbidity and Mortality Weekly Report Recommendation Report* 4: 54(RR–12): 1–81.

 [9] Bastian LA, Nanda K, Hasselblad V and Simel DL. 1998. Diagnostic efficiency of home pregnancy test kits. A meta-analysis. *Archives of Family Medicine.* 7(5): 465–469.

[10] Ariga R, Bloom K, Reddy VB, Kluskens L, Francescatti D, Dowlat K, Siziopikou K and Gattuso P. 2002. Fine-needle aspiration of clinically suspicious palpable breast masses with histopathologic correlation. *American Journal of Surgery.* **184**: 410–413.

[11] Johnson CA, Levey AS, Coresh J, Levin A, Lau J and Eknoyan G. 2004. Clinical Practice Guidelines for Chronic Kidney Disease in Adults: Part II. Glomerular Filtration Rate, Proteinuria, and Other Markers. *American Family Physician.* **70**: 1091–1097.

[12] Pelly TF, Santillan CF, Gilman RH, Cabrera LZ, Garcia E, Vidal C, Zimic MJ, Moore DA and Evans CA. 2005. Tuberculosis skin testing, anergy and protein malnutrition in Peru. *International Journal of Tuberculosis and Lung Diseases.* **9**(9): 977–984.

[13] Thompson IM and Ankerst DP. 2007. Prostate-specific antigen in the early detection of prostate cancer. *Canadian Medical Association Journal.* **176**(13): 1853–1858.

[14] How C. (ed). 2003. *Tuberculosis in Infancy and Childhood.* Philippine Pediatric Society Publications: Quezon City; pp 1–97.

[15] Parker C and Philp I. 2004. Screening for cognitive impairment among older people in black and minority ethnic groups. *Age and Ageing.* **33**(5): 447–452. Epub 2004 Jun 24.

[16] Steinbauer JR, Cantor SB, Holzer CE and Volk RJ. 1998. Ethnic and sex bias in primary care screening tests for alcohol use disorders. *Annals of Internal Medicine.* **129**(5): 353–362.

[17] Wong V, Hui LH, Lee WC, Leung LS, Ho PK, Lau WL, Fung CW and Chung B. 2004. A modified screening tool for autism (Checklist for Autism in Toddlers [CHAT-23]) for Chinese children. *Pediatrics.* **114**(2): 166–176.

[18] Glasziou P. 2001. Which methods for bedside Bayes? *Evidence Based Medicine.* **6**: 164–166.

[19] Otham S, Chia YC and Ng CJ. 2003. Accuracy of urinalysis in detection of urinary tract infection in a primary care setting. *Asia Pacific Family Medicine.* **2**(4): 206–212.

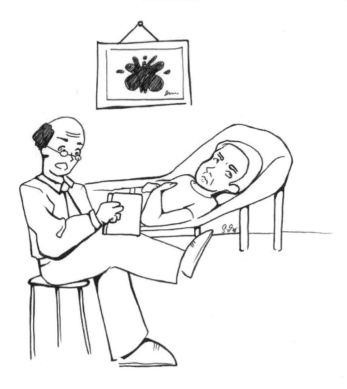

Well according to these tests you're feeling much better! Maybe you just don't know it yet...

4

Evaluation of Articles on Harm

Jacinto Blas V. Mantaring III, Antonio L. Dans, Felix Eduardo R. Punzalan

Studies on harm try to establish if a particular exposure is responsible for causing an undesirable outcome. Harmful exposures can be behaviours (e.g. tobacco or alcohol abuse), treatments (e.g. aspirin or warfarin intake) or patient characteristics (e.g. hypertension or exposure to pollution). In any of these situations, the questions on harm (or causation) should be phrased in terms of the following variables: P, the patient population that might be at risk; E, the potentially harmful exposures; and O, the outcomes that these exposures might cause. For example:

> Among healthy adults (P), how strongly associated is mobile phone use (E) with the risk of developing brain cancer (O)?

Painless Evidence-Based Medicine   Antonio L. Dans, Leonila F. Dans and Maria Asuncion A. Silvestre
© 2008 John Wiley & Sons, Ltd

4.1   Appraising directness

As in therapy and diagnosis, before reading an article on harm, we must first evaluate how well the PEO in the study (the research question) corresponds to our own PEO (your clinical question). Did the study recruit the types of patients you are interested in? Did they evaluate the exposure you are interested in? Even if the question is not exactly the same, sometimes the study can still provide some answers. For example, much of what we think we know about the effect of alcohol on health is derived from studies on red wine. The two exposures are not exactly the same, but whatever we learn about red wine can certainly provide some answers about the impact of alcohol intake in general. If you feel the article might help answer your question, then go ahead and evaluate it as in previous chapters.

4.2   Appraising validity

Question #1: Were the patient groups being compared sufficiently similar with respect to baseline characteristics? If not, were statistical adjustments made?

Perhaps the most important validity criterion which may influence the outcome of a harm study is the similarity in the baseline characteristics. How similar the groups are at the start of a study depends on which design was used, e.g. a randomized controlled trial, a cohort or a case-control study (see Tackle Box 4.1). Groups being compared are most similar in RCTs and least similar in case-control studies. When groups being compared are dissimilar, statisticians can make adjustments. These adjustments estimate what the study outcomes might have been had the baseline characteristics been the same. This may seem like salvaging data, and in fact this is what they are doing. However, this is the best we can do considering the imbalance inherent in some study designs.

Question #2: Were unbiased criteria used to determine exposure in all patients?

Ascertainment of the exposure is a key issue in studies on causation or harm. If ascertainment of exposure systematically favours one group compared to the other, it may lead us to a wrong estimate of the relationship between exposure and outcome. Determining exposure is not a problem in RCTs and cohort studies because exposure is either assigned (in RCTs) or carefully determined (in cohorts) at the start of the study.

Determining exposure is particularly problematic when we speak of case-control designs, as we often rely on the patients' ability to recall these exposures. This isn't a big problem if cases and controls had the same rates of recall as the difference would cancel out. Unfortunately, studies show that cases are more likely to recall an exposure than controls, probably because they already sustained an undesirable outcome[1]. This so-called 'recall bias' was demonstrated in a study where mothers were interviewed on likely causes of congenital anomalies in their offspring[2, 3]. Many years after a pregnancy, these mothers may be more likely to volunteer a prenatal history of cravings, medicines, exotic food, rituals, falls, etc. compared to mothers whose babies do not have anomalies.

Ascertainment of exposure in case-control studies may also be subject to bias on the part of the interviewer[4]. Interviewers may tend to be more persistent in their questioning for exposures among cases than controls. Readers should therefore look for strategies employed in the study to minimize this bias, such as blinding of interviewers.

Tackle Box 4.1 Three types of study designs used to evaluate the relationship between a potentially harmful exposure and an undesirable outcome

Instructions: Start going through this tackle box by understanding the diagrams in column 1. Once familiar with the diagrams and the basic differences in the designs, it will be easier to go through the columns on validity and feasibility.

Study design	Validity	Feasibility
Randomized controlled trial Patients → Randomize → Exposed → Outcome / No outcome → Unexposed → Outcome / No outcome	Highest validity. Baseline characteristics of exposed and unexposed tend to be very similar because of randomized assignment to these groups.	Lowest feasibility for three reasons: (1) If outcome is rare, a *big* sample size is required; (2) If prolonged exposure is necessary, long follow-up is required; (3) When exposure may be harmful, it may be unethical to randomize.
Cohort study Patients → Exposed → Outcome / No outcome → Unexposed → Outcome / No outcome	Midway in validity. Baseline characteristics of exposed and unexposed are rarely similar, but statisticians can make 'magical' adjustments.	Midway in feasibility. Budget is smaller because researchers don't need to pay for the exposure. Still, like RCTs, it may require a big sample size and prolonged follow-up.

| 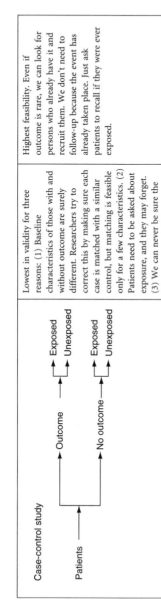 | Lowest in validity for three reasons: (1) Baseline characteristics of those with and without outcome are surely different. Researchers try to correct this by making sure each case is matched with a similar control, but matching is feasible only for a few characteristics. (2) Patients need to be asked about exposure, and they may forget. (3) We can never be sure the exposure preceded the outcome. | Highest feasibility. Even if outcome is rare, we can look for persons who already have it and recruit them. We don't need to follow-up because the event has already taken place. Just ask patients to recall if they were ever exposed. |

Case-control study

Notes:

1. Randomized controlled trials (discussed in Chapter 2) assign patients to either exposed (treated) or unexposed (untreated) groups who are then followed-up for a length of time to see how many do or don't develop outcomes.

2. Cohort studies are similar, except that we do not assign exposure. Patients come in and are already exposed or unexposed to a possibly harmful agent (by choice, e.g. when they smoke; or by chance, e.g. when they are born with genes for hypertension).

3. Case-control studies begin by recruiting patients with the outcome (*cases*) and without the outcome (*controls*), then proceed in the opposite direction by asking if they recall having been exposed to the harmful agent. For example, patients with lung cancer (cases) and without cancer (controls) may be asked whether they ever smoked or not.

Exercise: Design and implement a randomized controlled trial, a cohort and a case-control study on the harmful effects of smoking. In which one did you spend more?

Answers: Just kidding . . . but of course you'll spend more on your (unethical) RCT!

Question #3: Were unbiased criteria used to detect the outcome in all patients?

Detecting outcomes in study patients can be fraught with bias. This is not such a big problem in case-control studies because the outcome is determined at the start of the study and, in fact, is part of inclusion and exclusion criteria. In contrast, researchers conducting RCTs and cohort studies must pay special attention to ensure that outcome detection is unbiased. The best strategy to avoid this pitfall is to blind people tasked to ascertain outcome; they must not know if a particular patient is exposed or not.

Question #4: Was the follow-up rate adequate?

Cohorts and RCTs are generally conducted over a longer duration. Because of this, loss to follow-up is more often a problem than in case-control studies. Patients lost to follow-up may have suffered adverse events and because they have dropped out, we fail to incorporate their experiences in the analysis. Tackle Box 2.1 in Chapter 2 presents an approach to assessing if follow-up was adequate in a study. Essentially, readers should worry about dropouts if numbers are large enough to affect the outcome rates in a study.

4.3   Appraising the results

Question #1: How strong is the association between exposure and outcome?

In Tackle Box 2.2 of Chapter 2 we discussed various measures of effectiveness, such as the relative risk (RR), relative risk reduction (RRR), absolute risk reduction (ARR) and number needed to treat (NNT). These same measures also work for studies on harm designed as cohorts or RCTs. Instead of benefit, however, we will usually end up with values suggesting harm, i.e. RRR < 0, ARR < 0, RR > 1 and NNT < 0. Some people don't like numbers less than zero, so they omit the negative sign and just call them relative risk increase (RRI), absolute risk increase (ARI), or number needed to harm (NNH). It doesn't really matter as long as it is clear what the numbers represent. (If these numbers do not make sense, refer again to Tackle Box 2.2.)

For case-control studies, we use a slightly different measure of harm referred to as the *odds ratio* (OR). The odds ratio is read like a relative risk. A value more than 1 suggests harm (if OR = 2 then exposure doubles the odds of the outcome). A value less than 1 on the other hand, suggests benefit (if OR = 0.5 then exposure halves the odds of an outcome). Usually OR ~ RR, differing by only a few decimal places. To learn more of OR and RR, go through Tackle Box 4.2. If content with simply understanding the results or if seeing numbers causes you to break out in a rash, skip the tackle box and just move on!

Question #2: How precise is the estimate of the risk?

Just like RCTs on therapy, studies on harm merely estimate the true effect of an exposure. Thus, it may be unduly precise to express the OR as an exact point estimate (e.g. smoking causes cancer, OR = 14.0)[5]. As we pointed out in Chapter 2, point estimates such as these do not accurately reflect uncertainty in the studies that we do. Researchers therefore express the strength of an association as an 'interval estimate' which provides the range of possible values. Interval estimates are expressed at a 95% level of confidence. When we state 95% confidence intervals (95% CI), we mean that we are 95% sure that the true strength of association (the odds ratio) lies within this range. A better statement would therefore be 'smoking

Tackle Box 4.2   Why we measure odds ratios in case-control studies instead of relative risk

Instructions: A standard 2×2 table indicates (a) the exposure status in rows and (b) the outcome status in columns. Go through the 2×2 tables below to understand the difference between relative risk and odds ratio.

Panel A. 2×2 tables for RCTs and cohorts

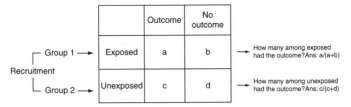

Panel B. 2×2 table for case-control studies

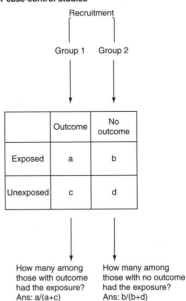

Notes:

1. Panel A demonstrates that sampling in RCTs and cohort studies is a horizontal event: we recruit exposed patients and follow them up to see the proportion who developed the outcomes. In this situation, it is rational to compare risk of outcomes in the exposed and unexposed, i.e. a/(a+b) ÷ c/(c+d). This is equivalent to the relative risk (RR) of an outcome (Chapter 2).

2. In contrast, the 2 × 2 table in Panel B shows that the sampling in case-controls is vertical: we recruit cases (persons with the outcome) and controls (persons without the outcome) and determine the proportion who were exposed. The rational comparison in this case would be risk of exposure among cases and the risk of exposure among controls, i.e. a/(a + c) ÷ b/(b + d). This may be referred to as the relative risk of an exposure. This would be a useless number. It would be like telling a patient: 'Sir, you have lung cancer, there is a 10-fold rise in the risk that you are a smoker'!

3. To counter this problem, statisticians use the *odds* of exposure a/c ('a is to c') and b/d ('b is to d') instead of the *risk* of the exposure which is a/(a + c) and b/(b + d). (You might want to review Tackle Box 3.2, if you find this confusing.) The ratio of odds would then be (a/c) ÷ (b/d). This is still a vertical comparison. Instead of the useless relative risk of exposure, we have converted it to a useless relative odds of exposure. Or 'Sir, you have lung cancer, there is a 10-fold rise in the *odds* that you are a smoker'! However, this vertical 'odds ratio' (OR) has four advantages over the relative risk (RR): (a) it is equivalent to the horizontal odds ratio (a/b) ÷ (c/d), which is our main interest or 'Sir, you are a smoker, so your odds of having lung cancer is 10 times higher'; (b) numerically, the OR is almost the same as the relative risk, usually differing by only a few decimal places; (c) it can be reduced to a ridiculously simple equation OR = ad/bc and (d) it not only works for just case-control studies, it will also work for RCTs and cohorts.

Exercise: If a = 4, b = 21, c = 1, d = 24, compute (a) the relative risk; (b) the odds ratio.

Answers: RR = 4.0; OR = 4.6

increases the risk of lung cancer 14-fold, but it could range somewhere between a 3-fold and 59-fold increase'[5]. By convention, this is expressed in the following syntax:

$$OR = 14.0 \ [95\% \ CI : 3.3, 59.3]$$

How do we interpret the 95% CI? Recall the four basic tenets for therapy:

1. When both ends of the CI are on the side of benefit (OR < 1), the exposure definitely reduces the odds of the unfavourable outcome.
2. When both ends of the CI are on the side of harm (OR > 1), the exposure definitely increases the odds of the unfavourable outcome.
3. When one end reflects an important reduction in odds and the other end reflects an important increase in odds, the study is inconclusive.
4. When one end reflects a small unimportant reduction in odds and the other end reflects a small unimportant increase in odds, then for all intents and purposes the exposure has no effect on the outcome.

Confused? Then, you may need to review Tackle Box 2.3 in Chapter 2. This will be time well spent, because it will help you analyse study results quickly and efficiently!

4.4   Assessing applicability

Now that we have appraised the validity and the results of the article, we can decide if the results apply to your own patient. As in previous chapters, we suggest two things to consider when studying applicability: biologic and socioeconomic issues.

Biologic issues affecting applicability

Biologic factors may affect the applicability of a study on harm to your particular patient. These biologic issues include differences in sex, co-morbidity, race, age and pathology.

Sex

Consider physiological, hormonal or biochemical differences between sexes that may impact on the effect of an exposure on the outcome. Heavy smoking increases the risk of oral cancer in men, with an OR = 2.1 [95% CI: 1.4, 3.2]. In women, the OR is 4.6 [95% CI: 2.5, 8.7][6].

Co-morbidities

Consider co-existing conditions that could affect the risk of an outcome for a given exposure. Chronic rofecoxib use increases the risk of cardiovascular events overall. Among patients with indications for ASA, the OR is 4.89 [95% CI: 1.41, 16.88]. Among patients with no indication for ASA, the OR is only 1.89 [95% CI: 1.03, 3.45][7].

Race

Consider racial or ethnic differences that may alter the risk for the outcome. Angiotensin-Converting Enzyme (ACE) inhibitors (a class of antihypertensives) increase the risk of angioedema. The risk is three times higher in blacks than in whites[8]. The odds of developing hepatitis with isoniazid use is lower among Asians who are fast acetylators of the drug[9].

Age

Consider the age of the population in the study in relation to the population that you are interested in. Inhaled corticosteroids increase the risk for cataracts in asthmatic patients older than 40 years of age, but not in younger patients[10].

Pathology

Diseases referred to by the same name may sometimes represent pathologic states that differ in subtle ways. These differences may sometimes account for variations in predisposition to disease. For example, the relationship between high salt intake and hypertension is stronger among blacks. This is probably caused by a higher prevalence of salt sensitivity[11].

Socioeconomic factors affecting applicability

Socioeconomic status is known to modify the relationship between exposure and outcome for a wide variety of conditions. This applies to many infectious diseases that afflict low to middle-income countries all over the world (such as tuberculosis, malaria and diarrhoea). However, socioeconomic status can also affect causation of several chronic degenerative diseases. For example, the OR for developing peptic ulcer disease from *H. pylori* infection in Denmark is 1.6 [95% CI: 0.8, 3.4] in higher socioeconomic classes, compared to 4.1 [95% CI: 1.8, 9.2] in lower socioeconomic classes[12]. It also affects the relationship between smoking, alcohol, diet and oesophageal cancer[13], smoking and chronic obstructive lung disease[14], diabetes and stroke[15], and many other diseases.

4.5   Individualizing the results

If you feel that the biologic and socioeconomic factors do not significantly limit applicability, you can proceed to individualize the estimate of harm. Studies report the average effect of exposure in the population. However, the magnitude of this effect will vary slightly between patients. The main source of variation is the patient's baseline risk for the adverse outcome. Variation in risk is very common in medicine. Patients have mild, moderate or severe forms of the same disease, or may have different risk factors for an adverse outcome. Some may come in early, and others may come in late in the course of an illness. Tackle Box 4.3 shows us four quick steps in using the baseline risk to estimate the effect of the exposure on an individual.

4.6 Summary

Studies on harm help us decide whether or not to avoid a certain exposure. Sometimes these studies lead us to avoid certain behaviours (e.g. smoking or alcoholism) or certain treatments. To read articles on harm efficiently, start by evaluating how directly they answer questions that are important to you. If the patients, exposures or outcomes are similar to those you are interested in, go ahead and assess validity. Bear in mind that our hands are often tied when we study harm, because the ideal study (an RCT) would be too long, too large or even unethical.

After appraising validity, appraise the results. Don't get bogged down with numbers and computations. Most of the time, the authors tell you what the ORs and RRs are (excuse the tongue twister). Of course, just as in articles on therapy and diagnosis, you must next assess applicability, because biologic and socio-economic factors may affect relationships between risk factors and outcomes.

Lastly, you can proceed to individualize the results and estimate risks specific to your patient, that is, the patients absolute risk increase and NNH. Again, don't get too engrossed with numerical sophistication if this is difficult for you. ORs and RRs are nothing more than estimates of how exposure changes risk, expressed as a multiple of the baseline risk.

Tackle Box 4.3   Estimating impact of a harmful exposure on individual patients

Instructions: The effect of an exposure on the risk of disease varies from individual to individual. This variation can be attributed to differences in the baseline risk for a disease. Go through this Tackle Box in rows, from step 1 to step 4, to understand the process involved in individualizing risk. In the rightmost column, we have a running example of a hypertensive woman considering the possibility of harm if she takes phenylpropanolamine (PPA) for her colds.

Step	How to do this	Need an equation?
Step 1: Estimate the baseline risk or pre-exposure risk in percent.	If the article you are reading is a cohort study, it may already contain this information. Look for a subgroup of unexposed individuals that closely approximates the one you are seeing. If the study does not contain this information, you might need to look at community-based studies.	There isn't any . . . Example: Let's say we have a patient with BP of 220/120. Studies show that the baseline risk for a haemorrhagic stroke is high, about 6% per year[16].
Step 2: Convert baseline risk to baseline odds.	Risk is usually expressed as a probability. Probabilities are portions of the whole, while odds are the ratio of portions. Say that again? Well, if we were talking of a pie, probability would be a piece of the pie divided by the entire pie. Odds, on the other hand, would be a piece of the pie divided by the rest of pie. To convert from probability to odds, we simply reduce the denominator by subtracting the numerator from it. For example, 7/100 (probability) becomes 7/93 (odds); 92/100 (probability) becomes 92/8 (odds)*.	$$Odds = \frac{Probability(\%)}{100 - Probability(\%)}$$ Example: If the risk of a haemorrhagic stroke is 6%, the odds will be 6/94.

Step 3: Multiply baseline odds by the Odds Ratio to get the post-exposure odds.	The baseline odds are derived in step 2. The study you read should tell you the OR of the exposure. Remember, a harmful exposure will probably have an OR > 1.0. Thus, an OR of 2 doubles the odds of an event!	Post-exposure odds = Baseline $odds \times OR$ Example: Exposure to PPA increases the risk of haemorrhagic stroke with OR ~2.0[17]; the post-exposure risk in our example is therefore 2 × 6/94 or 12/94.
Step 4: Convert post-exposure odds to post-exposure risk in percent.	Simple. Just add the numerator back to the denominator. For example, 1/3 (odds) becomes 1/4 (probability) and 0.24 (odds) becomes 0.24/1.24 (probability). This is now your patient's risk after exposure!	$$Probability = \frac{Odds}{1 + Odds} \times 100$$ Example: If odds are 12/94, then the probability is 12/106 or about 11.3%. If we use the formula above, 12/94 = 0.128, so probability is (0.128/1.128)×100 = 11.3%.

Notes:

1. You can skip converting probabilities to odds (step 2) and odds to probabilities (step 4) in situations when: (a) the baseline risk is very small because for all intents and purposes, odds and probability will be equal (e.g. if the probability is 1/100, odds will be 1/99, an ignorable difference); and (b) the measure of risk is expressed as a 'relative risk' rather than an odds ratio. In both these situations, all you need to do is multiply baseline risk by the OR or RR.

2. Once you have the pre-exposure and post-exposure risk, you can do a lot of patient-specific calculations! (a) Post-exposure risk minus baseline risk = individualized absolute risk increase (ARI). In the example above, 11.3% – 6% = 5.3%. (b) 100/(absolute risk increase) = individualized number needed to harm (NNH). In the example above, 100/5.3 = 19.

3. Individualized information can now be used to guide a decision on whether or not to avoid a potentially harmful exposure.

Exercise: If the baseline risk for stroke was 1% in the example above, what would be the ARI and NNH for stroke if the patient received PPA?

Answer: ARI = 1%, NNH = 100

⋆ *Déjà vu* – a feeling of tedious familiarity.

References

[1] Delgado-Rodríguez M and Llorca J. 2004. Bias. *Journal of Epidemiology and Community Health*. **58**: 635–641.

[2] Werler MM, Pober BR, Nelson K and Holmes LB. 1989. Reporting accuracy among mothers of malformed and non-malformed infants. *American Journal of Epidemiology*. **129**(2): 415–421.

[3] Rockenbauer M, Olsen J, Czeizel AE, Pedersen L, Sorensen, Henrik T and the EuroMAP Group. 2001. Recall bias in a case-control surveillance system on the use of medicine during pregnancy. *Epidemiology*. **12**(4): 461–466.

[4] Blomgren KJ, Sundstrom A, Steineck G and Wilholm BE. 2006. Interviewer variability – quality aspects in a case-control study. *European Journal of Epidemiology*. **21**(4): 267–277.

[5] Doll R and Hill AB. 1950. Smoking and carcinoma of the lung. Preliminary report. *British Medical Journal*. **2**: 739–748.

[6] Muscat JE, Richie JP Jr, Thompson S and Wynder EL. 1996. Gender differences in smoking and risk for oral cancer. *Cancer Research*. **1556**(22): 5192–5197.

[7] Mukherjee D, Nissen SE and Topol EJ. 2001. Risk of cardiovascular events with selective COX-2 inhibitors. *Journal of American Medical Association*. **286**(8): 954–959.

[8] Kostis JB, Kim HJ, Rusnak J, Casale T, Kaplan A, Corren J and Levy E. 2005. Incidence and characteristics of angioedema associated with enalapril. *Archives of Internal Medicine*. **165**(14): 1637–1642.

[9] Huang YS, Chern HD, Su WJ, Lai SL, Yang SY, Chang FY and Lee SD. 2002. Polymorphism of the N-acetyltransferase gene as a susceptibility risk factor for antituberculosis drug-induced hepatitis. *Hepatology*. **35**(4): 883–889.

[10] Jick SS, Vasilakis-Scaramozza C and Maier WC. 2001. The risk of cataract among users of inhaled steroids. *Epidemiology*. **12**(2): 229–234.

[11] Wilson DK, Bayer L and Sica DA. 1996. Variability in saly sensitivity classification in black male versus female adolescents. *Hypertension*. **28**(2): 250–255.

[12] Rosenstock SJ, Jorgensen T, Bonnevie O and Andersen P. 2004. Does *Helicobacter pylori* infection explain all socioeconomic differences in peptic ulcer incidence? Genetic and psychosocial markers for incident peptic ulcer disease in a large cohort of Danish adults. *Scandinavian Journal of Gastroenterology*. **39**(9): 823–829.

[13] Wu M, Zhao JK, Hu XS, Wang PH, Qin Y, Lu YC, Yang J, Liu AM, Wu DL, Zhang ZF, Frans KJ and van't Veer P. 2006. Association of smoking, alcohol drinking and dietary factors with esophageal cancer in high- and low-risk areas of Jiangsu Province, China. *World Journal of Gastroenterology.* **12**(11): 1686–1693.

[14] Thorn J, Björkelund C, Bengtsson C, Guo X, Lissner L and Sundh V. 2006. Low socio-economic status, smoking, mental stress and obesity predict obstructive symptoms in women, but only smoking also predicts subsequent experience of poor health. *International Journal Medical Science.* **34**(1): 7–12.

[15] Avendano M, Kawachi I, Van Lenthe F, Boshuizen HC, Mackenbach JP, Van den Bos GA, Fay ME and Berkman LF. 2006. Socioeconomic status and stroke incidence in the US elderly: the role of risk factors in the EPESE study. *Stroke.* **37**(6): 1368–1373. Epub 2006 May 11.

[16] Song Y, Sung J, Lawlor DA, Smith GD, Shin Y and Ebrahim S. 2004. Blood pressure, haemorrhagic stroke, and ischaemic stroke: the Korean national prospective occupational cohort study. *British Medical Journal.* **328**: 324–325.

[17] Kernan WN, Viscoli CM, Brass LM, Broderick JP, Brott T, Feldmann E, Morgenstern LB, Wilterdink JL and Horwitz, RI. 2000. Phenyl-propanolamine and the risk of haemorrhagic stroke. *New England Journal of Medicine.* **343**(25): 1826–1832.

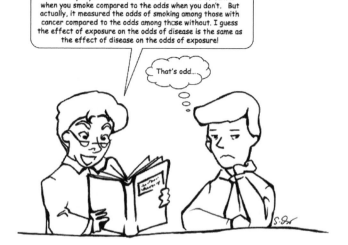

5

Evaluation of Articles on Prognosis

Felix Eduardo R. Punzalan, Antonio L. Dans, Jacinto Blas V. Mantaring III, Leonila F. Dans

People with a disease have important questions about how their particular condition will affect their lives. Patients and their families want to know what to expect. What is the chance of dying from the disease? What are its complications? How often do they occur? Studies on prognosis evaluate the likelihood of outcomes developing over time in patients with a particular clinical condition. This information helps patients make important decisions about their own healthcare.

5.1 Appraising directness

A clinical question on prognosis is usually phrased using the variables P, the patient or population with a certain disease and O, the outcome or complication of interest. For example,

Painless Evidence-Based Medicine   Antonio L. Dans, Leonila F. Dans and Maria Asuncion A. Silvestre
© 2008 John Wiley & Sons, Ltd

> Among patients with angina (P), what is the likelihood of developing myocardial infarction (O)?

Sometimes, we are interested in how certain characteristics of the population affect prognosis. In this case, we also refer to a variable E, an exposure or 'prognostic factor' that affects risk of an outcome. For example,

> Among patients with diabetes mellitus (P), how does the presence of proteinuria (E) affect the likelihood of developing renal failure (O)?

The usual design for answering this question is a cohort study (see Tackle Box 4.1) where patients with the condition are followed up for a certain duration to measure the frequency of occurrence of the outcome. As before, begin appraising an article on prognosis by deciding if it provides a direct enough answer to the question you are asking. Pay particular attention to the population (P) because even when the disease is the same, prognosis can vary greatly depending on subtype, severity and stage of disease. If you think the patients in the study (or subgroups of them) are similar enough to the patient you are seeing, appraise validity. Otherwise, look for an article that gives you a closer answer to the question you ask.

5.2 Appraising validity

Question #1: Was the sample of patients representative?

Ensure that the population of patients recruited by the study is representative of the patients with the condition in question. If the authors claim to estimate stroke rates among patients with hypertension in general, recruiting hypertensives admitted to a hospital would surely lead to an inappropriately morbid prediction. If they claim to measure stroke rates among hypertensives admitted to a hospital, then recruiting confined patients would be appropriate. To evaluate how representative a study is, examine the research objective. If you feel the inclusion and exclusion criteria are appropriate to the population (P) that they address then the sample of patients is probably representative.

Question #2: Were patients (or subgroups of patients) sufficiently homogeneous with respect to prognostic risk?

The prognosis of most diseases is determined by characteristics of the patient (e.g. age, sex and state of nutrition) and characteristics of the disease (e.g. stage, subtype and duration). Because of this, many times, it may not make sense to simply make an overall average prognosis. Such an average risk would overestimate risk in patients with mild disease and underestimate risk in patients with severe illness.

A more valid approach to summarizing results would be to group patients according to the presence or absence of the aforementioned prognostic factors. For example, a study on the survival of patients with congestive heart failure might subgroup patients according to age, functional class and even etiology of heart failure (ischemic *versus* idiopathic).

Deciding whether groups in a study are sufficiently homogeneous can be tricky. One must have clinical experience or knowledge of the disease biology to decide if there are other prognostic factors that the authors may have failed to consider.

Question #3: Were unbiased criteria used to detect the outcome in all patients?

Outcomes may be classified by the degree of objectivity needed to classify them. *Hard* outcomes are those that require little judgment to ascertain, e.g. the *fact* of death. *Soft* outcomes, on the other hand, require subjective judgment, e.g. the *cause* of death, or quality of life. The softer the outcome, the more important it is to define criteria on which they can be based. Researchers spend a lot of energy defining outcomes, even if it seems (on the surface) to be easily determined. Myocardial infarction, for example, was defined in a study as follows:

> A diagnosis of myocardial infarction was made if the following conditions were met: creatine kinase or creatine kinase-MB more than twice the upper limit of normal; or troponin I or T more than twice the upper limit of normal (if neither creatine kinase or creatine kinase-MB were available); or troponin I or T more than three times the upper limit of normal for the same markers within 24 h of percutaneous transluminal coronary angioplasty; or troponin I or T more than five times the upper limit of normal for the same markers within 24 h of coronary artery bypass grafting surgery. In addition to these marker criteria, a patient had to have experienced electrocardiographic changes in two or more contiguous leads showing new Q waves (or R waves in V1 or V2), left bundle branch block, or ischaemic ST-T wave changes, or typical clinical presentation consistent with myocardial infarction defined as one of the following: cardiac ischaemic-type pain lasting more than 20 min, pulmonary oedema, or cardiogenic shock not otherwise explained[1].

Whew, talk about complex definitions! The more subjective the interpretation, the more detailed the criteria we need. Moreover, even after we go through the complexities of a definition such as this, we need to protect implementation of these criteria, by blinding those who will use them. As we discussed in Chapter 2, prior expectations on outcomes can sway decisions about whether the outcomes actually occurred or not.

Question #4: Was follow-up rate adequate?

Prognosticating is about knowing the likelihood of an outcome. Therefore, having patients whose outcomes are unknown because they failed to follow-up makes the estimate of prognosis less certain. The higher the proportion of those who were lost to follow-up, the greater is the threat to validity. This becomes even more worrisome when you suspect that an adverse event is more likely among patients who drop out from the study.

Just as in articles on therapy, the crucial issue is ascertaining when you should worry about the number of drop-outs. This should be relatively simple for articles on prognosis. Simply assume the worst event for the drop-outs, add them to the overall event rate and see if this significantly changes the conclusions. If the change in the conclusions is significant, then there were too many drop-outs.

5.3 Appraising the results

Question #1: How likely are the outcomes over time?

The results from studies about prognosis can be expressed in pictures or in numbers. Common numbers used are the 1. event rate; 2. event-free rate; and 3. average time to an event.

These are discussed in Table 5.1.

Reporting prognosis in pictures is even more informative. If you are familiar with survival curves, you can skip Tackle Box 5.1 altogether. If not, please spend some time on it before proceeding.

Question #2: How precise are the estimates of likelihood?

When presented as numbers (event-free rates, event rates or average survival), the likelihood of an outcome can be expressed

Table 5.1 Reporting prognosis in numbers

Expression of prognosis	Definition	Example
Event rate	Percentage of patients who have the undesirable outcome over time	Mortality rate, stroke rate, hospitalization rate
Event-free rate	Percentage of patients who do not have the outcome over time	Survival rate, stroke-free survival rate, pain-free survival rate
Average survival	Average length of time before an event occurs	Mean survival, median survival, average time to event

with a range of possibilities known as 95% Confidence Intervals (CIs). The interval gives us the best and worst scenarios in terms of prognosis of the condition being evaluated. The narrower the confidence interval, the more precise is the estimate.

When presented as survival curves, these 95% CIs can be shown at specific points in the graph as shown in Figure 5.1. Usually the survival curves are more precise in the earlier periods of a study since it includes more patients. As the study goes on, patients are lost to follow-up and the 95% CIs become wider.

5.4 Assessing applicability

Biologic issues affecting applicability

As in previous chapters, applicability of findings of studies on prognosis can be affected by biologic factors that include sex, co-morbid conditions, race, age and pathology.

Tackle Box 5.1   Reporting prognosis in pictures

Instructions: The results of prognosis studies are often reported in survival curves. Usually, the x-axis represents time and the y-axis is scaled from 100% survival (top) to 0% survival (at the bottom). Go through this tackle box to learn more about interpreting survival curves.

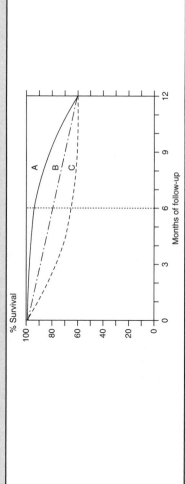

Notes:
1. Survival curves give us more information than simple numbers depicting overall rates. Compare the three survival curves above. Despite a similar overall survival rate of 60% after 12 months of follow-up, there is a distinct survival advantage for line A. By the sixth month, more than 90% of patients in line A had survived, but for line C, survival was only a little over 60%. Patients in line B lie somewhere in between. As you can see, the curves tell a more accurate story than the overall survival rates.

2. If we're interested in events other than death, we can rename the x-axis as a generic 'event-free survival'. We can also be more specific and state the exact event: for example, pain-free survival or stroke-free survival.

3. Some authors prefer using event rates, instead of event-free survival. In this case, the curves would start from 0 events at the bottom of the x-axis, and gradually go up through time: an exact mirror image of a survival curve. Figure 2.1 is an example of such a graph.

Exercise: Which of the above three curves illustrates the best survival rate in the first six months?
Answer: Curve A

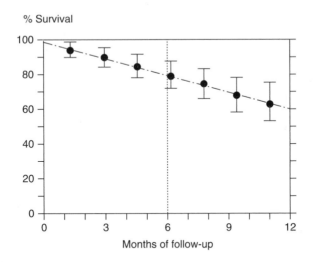

Figure 5.1 Survival rates over a 12-month follow-up period

Sex

Consider sex differences that alter disease prognosis. For example, in-hospital mortality after coronary artery bypass surgery is two times higher in women than in men[2].

Co-morbid conditions

Consider other clinical conditions that may alter prognosis. High in-hospital mortality has been noted among Filipinos after a myocardial infarction[3]. This has been partially attributed to a higher incidence of hospital-acquired pneumonia among those admitted in government facilities. Similarly, it has been noted that concomitant hypertension is an independent predictor of progression to kidney failure among diabetic patients[4].

Race

Ethnic or racial factors are another important determinant of prognosis in many conditions. Asians, for example, have a slightly lower risk of deep vein thrombosis after major orthopaedic surgery[5]. Similarly, African-American women have higher mortality after breast cancer than white women[6].

Age

Age is an important prognostic factor in almost any condition. For example, shorter survival times with recurrent breast cancer are predicted in women of ages younger than 35 years (irrespective of menopausal status)[7]. Survival is also significantly lower for children with ependymoma who are less than 4 years of age[8]. On the other hand, older females with cervical cancer[9] and advanced ovarian cancer[10] have poorer survival.

Pathology

Consider factors relating to disease severity, stage or subtype, because these are the main determinants of disease progression. The medical literature is replete with examples. The more severe the BP elevation, the higher is the risk of stroke. The more extensive the infection, the more catastrophic is its course. The more malignant the histology, the earlier is the metastasis.

Socioeconomic issues affecting applicability

Socioeconomic conditions may affect prognosis, especially when prognosis is highly dependent on the quality of medical care that patients receive. In a study among Filipinos with acute MI, in-hospital mortality was two times higher in patients admitted to a charity government hospital when compared to private hospitals. This was partially attributed to the limited availability of costly thrombolytic agents[3]. In a cohort study of elderly patients with prostate carcinoma, it was shown that low socioeconomic status was significantly associated with decreasing survival even after adjustment for age, co-morbidity and treatment. Those living in the community within the lowest quartile of socioeconomic status were 31% more likely to die than those living in the highest quartile[11].

Inevitably, some differences will arise and your patient will not always be similar to the study patient. You should assess whether the study patients are so different from yours that you cannot confidently use the results in making predictions for your patients. If there are no burning biologic or socioeconomic issues that limit the applicability of the study, you can use the study results for prognostic information.

5.5 Individualizing the results

The more variables found to affect outcome, the more difficult it becomes to estimate the risk of an individual patient. To estimate the annual risk of a coronary event in an individual, for example, one would need to consider age, sex, family history, blood pressure, waist-to-hip ratio, serum cholesterol, blood sugar and even socioeconomic status. Because these calculations present with so many variables, some researchers have developed risk equations and scoring systems in an attempt to simplify the task of risk stratification. Thus, Goldman's score estimates the risk of life-threatening complications after non-cardiac surgery[12] and the Apache score is used to estimate mortality risk after admission to the intensive care unit of critically ill cancer patients[13]. Some have even gone to the extent of developing electronic calculators that do all the mathematics for us: for example, the Framingham risk calculator[14]. The main goal in using these various instruments is to come up with an estimate of prognosis specific to an individual patient, based on that individual's characteristics. This information is useful in making treatment decisions.

Prognostic data is also used to inform a patient, about what to expect of their condition. This is always an important aspect of management. A valid prognostic study may not alter treatment decisions; however, it can always give the patient a glimpse of the future.

5.6 Summary

Information on disease prognosis helps us to decide whether we want to treat an illness or just leave it alone. In addition, however, estimates of prognosis may be used as baseline risks for our patients when we try to individualize the results of treatment (see Chapter 2) or harm (see Chapter 4).

As usual, begin evaluation of the article by deciding whether it provides a direct answer to the question you ask. Only then should you spend time going deeper. Validity can be appraised quickly by checking on four criteria: how representative the study is, homogeneity of study subjects, objectivity of outcomes and completeness of follow-up. When satisfied that the study is valid, interpret the results. These can be presented as numbers (disease-free survival rate, event rates, or mean time to event) or as graphs (disease-free survival curves or curves of cumulative events). Before using the numbers on your patient, ensure that biologic and socioeconomic factors will not limit applicability of the results. Finally, try to come up with a risk estimate that is specific for your patient. Check subgroups in the study that your patient might fit into. If there are too many, look for a scoring system that the authors might have provided.

References

[1] Pfeffer MA, Swedberg K, Granger CB, Held P, McMurray JJ, Michelson EL, Olofsson B, Ostergren J, Yusuf J, Pocock S and CHARM Investigators and Committees. 2003. Effects of candesartan on mortality and morbidity in patients with chronic heart failure: the CHARM-Overall programme. *Lancet*. **362**: 759–766.

[2] Hannan EL, Wu C, Bennett EV, Carlson RE, Culliford AT, Gold JP, Higgins RSD, Isom OW, Smith CR, and Jones RH. 2006. Risk stratification of in-hospital mortality for coronary artery bypass graft surgery. *Journal of American College of Cardiology*. **47**: 661–668.

[3] The Isip Study Group. 1999. Acute myocardial infarction in tertiary centers in Metro Manila: In-hospital survival and physicians practices. Infarct survival in the Philippines: In-hospital mortality (ISIP). *Asean Heart Journal*. **7**(1): 1–7.

[4] Bruno G, Biggeri A, Merletti F, Bargero G, Ferrero S, Pagano G and Perin PC. 2003. Low incidence of end-stage renal disease and chronic renal failure in type 2 diabetes: 10 year prospective study. *Diabetes Care*. **26**(8): 2353–2358.

[5] Leizorovicz A, Turpie AGG, Cohen AT, Wong L, Yoo MC and Dans A for the SMART Study Group. 2005. Epidemiology of venous thromboembolism in Asian patients undergoing major orthopedic surgery without thromboprophylaxis. The SMART Study. *Journal of Thrombosis and Haemostatis*. **3**: 28–34.

[6] Chlebowski RT, Chen Z, Anderson GL, Rohan T, Aragaki A, Lane D, Dolan NC, Paskett ED, McTiernan A, Hubbell A, Adams-Campbell LL, Prentice R. 2005. Ethnicity and breast cancer: factors influencing differences in incidence and outcome. *Journal of National Cancer Institute*. **97**(6): 439–448.

[7] Falkson G, Gelman RS and Pretorius FJ. 1986. Age as a prognostic factor in recurrent breast cancer. *Journal of Clinical Oncology*. **4**: 663–671.

[8] Sala F, Talacchi A, Mazza C, Prisco R, Ghimenton C and Bricolo A. 1998. Prognostic factors in childhood intracranial ependymomas: The role of age and tumor location. *Pediatric Neurosurgery*. **28**: 135–142.

[9] Meanwell CA, Kelly KA, Wilson S, Roginski C, Woodman C, Griffiths R and Blackledge G. 1988. Young age as a prognostic factor in cervical cancer: analysis of population based data from 10 022 cases. *British Medical Journal*. **296**(6619): 386–391.

[10] Thigpen T, Brady MF, Omura GA, Creasman WT, McGuire WP, Hoskins WJ and Williams S. 1993. Age as a prognostic factor in ovarian carcinoma. The Gynecologic Oncology Group experience. *Cancer*. **71**(2 Suppl): 606–614.

[11] Du XL, Fang S, Coker AL, Sanderson M, Aragaki C, Cormier JN, Xing Y, Gor BJ and Chan W. 2006. Racial disparity and socioeconomic status in association with survival in older men with local/regional stage prostate carcinoma: findings from a large community-based cohort. *Cancer*. **106**(6): 1276–1285.

[12] Prause G, Ratzenhofer-Comenda B, Pierer G, Smolle-Juttner F, Glanzer H and Smolle J. 1997. Can ASA grade or Goldman's cardiac risk index predict peri-operative mortality? A study of 16,227 patients. *Anaesthesia*. **52**(3): 203–206.

[13] Chang L, Horng CF, Huang YC and Hsieh YY. 2006. Prognostic accuracy of acute physiology and chronic health evaluation II scores in critically ill cancer patients. *American Journal of Critical Care*. **15**(1): 47–53.

[14] http://hp2010.nhlbihin.net/atpiii/calculator.asp

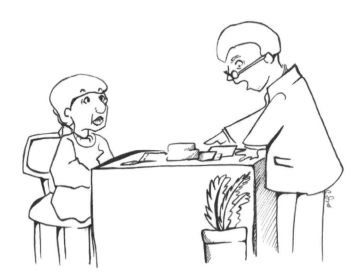

'There's something wrong Mrs. Cruz. We need to do more tests. According to this study you should have had a stroke a year ago!'

6

Evaluation of Systematic Reviews

Marissa M. Alejandria, Bernadette A. Tumanan-Mendoza, Ma. Vanessa Villarruz-Sulit, Antonio L. Dans

So far, we have breezed through the appraisal of four common types of articles encountered in medicine: articles on therapy, diagnosis, prognosis and harm. The last type of article to be discussed in this book is the systematic review. A systematic review summarizes the results of several studies that seem to answer the same clinical question. It is distinguished from traditional *reviews*, by the use of systematic methods to

1. identify, select and critically appraise relevant studies; and

2. collect and analyse data from the included studies to minimize bias[1].

A systematic review may use statistical methods to summarize the results of included studies. In this case, it is referred to as a 'meta-analysis'.

Painless Evidence-Based Medicine   Antonio L. Dans, Leonila F. Dans and Maria Asuncion A. Silvestre
© 2008 John Wiley & Sons, Ltd

Authors conduct systematic reviews to

1. draw a reliable conclusion based on a summary of all relevant studies;

2. increase the precision of estimates of the effectiveness of treatment, accuracy of tests, magnitude of risk and prognosis of disease;

3. increase the number of patients in clinically relevant subgroups;

4. resolve uncertainty when results of primary studies seem conflicting; and

5. plan new studies when there is lack of adequate evidence.

6.1   Appraising directness

Systematic reviews are usually conducted to summarize several articles on therapy, but they may also be used to answer questions on diagnosis, prognosis or harm. We begin to analyse a systematic review by appraising how directly it addresses the question raised, i.e. how well the PEO in the study corresponds to our own PEO. The issue of directness of studies on therapy, diagnosis, harm and prognosis has been discussed in detail in Chapters 2–5. When we look at systematic reviews on this topic, however, a unique issue arises: the sensibility of the research question. Some questions are so broad that they do not really correspond to the interest of health care providers and patients. An example of an overly broad question is:

> Among patients with cancer, how effective is chemotherapy in delaying disease progression?

In this example, there are too many different cancers and chemotherapeutic agents. Combining the results of these various studies would not yield a meaningful estimate of effectiveness. To make this question sensible, we need to focus them so they refer to a specific population, exposure and outcome. For example, among older women with operable breast cancer (a specific cancer population), how effective is tamoxifen (a specific chemotherapeutic agent) in prolonging survival (a specific outcome).

If you feel the article provides a reasonably direct answer and that the reviewers pose a sensible question, then proceed to read it in more detail. Otherwise, look for a better paper.

6.2 Appraising validity

Question #1: Were the criteria for inclusion of studies appropriate?

While primary studies describe criteria for inclusion or exclusion of individual *patients*, systematic reviews describe criteria for inclusion or exclusion of individual *studies*. These criteria describe the methodological quality of the studies (M) to be included, as well as the populations (P), exposures (E) and outcomes (O)[2]. In the hierarchy of evidence, randomized controlled trials (RCTs) come with the least bias, followed by cohort studies, case-control studies and surveys. The lowest in the hierarchy would be descriptive studies including case series and single case reports.

The type of study design to be included in a systematic review depends on the type of clinical question the review is addressing. Of course, the best study design may not always be available for a certain question. In this case, reviewers should be less rigid in their inclusion criteria in order to accommodate study designs of lower validity.

Question #2: Was the search for eligible studies thorough?

A comprehensive search of the literature is important to ensure that relevant studies, both published and unpublished, are not missed. A thorough search for published literature should include use of electronic medical databases such as MEDLINE, EMBASE, the Cochrane Library and non-English language databases. Cross-references of original publications are also a good source of published articles.

One problem with literature searches is that studies that report a 'positive' result are more likely to be published than 'negative' studies. Thus, if only published articles are sought, conclusions may overestimate the effectiveness of an intervention, safety of a therapy or the accuracy of a test. This phenomenon has been well-documented and is often referred to as 'publication bias'[3].

Avoiding publication bias in systematic reviews entails a thorough search for unpublished articles. This may be done by writing to experts, going through pharmaceutical industry files or surveying conference proceedings and books of abstracts. Among other sources, unpublished trials can now be found in the WHO Network of Collaborating Clinical Trial Registers, Clinical-Trials.gov from the US National Institutes of Health, the US Food and Drug Administration (FDA) registry, and the International Committee of Medical Journal Editors (ICMJE) registry[4].

Question #3: Was the validity of the included studies assessed?

Look for an assessment of the methodological quality of the included studies in the review. Check whether the authors used validity criteria for appraising primary studies (similar to those presented in preceding chapters). For example, in a systematic

Table 6.1 Important validity criteria for assessing the quality of primary studies included in a systematic review

Study Type	Validity Criteria
Therapy	Were patients randomly assigned to treatment groups?
	Was allocation concealed?
	Were baseline characteristics similar at the start of the trial?
	Were patients blinded to the treatment assignment?
	Were caregivers blinded to treatment assignment?
	Were outcome assessors blinded to the treatment assignment?
	Were all patients analysed in the groups they were originally randomized?
	Was follow-up rate adequate?
Diagnosis	Was the reference standard an acceptable one?
	Was the reference standard interpreted independently from the test in question?
Harm or causation	Were the patient groups being compared sufficiently similar with respect to baseline characteristics?
	If not, were statistical adjustments made?
	Were unbiased criteria used to determine exposure in all patients?
	Were unbiased criteria used to detect the outcome in all patients?
	Was follow-up rate adequate?
Prognosis	Was the sample of patients representative?
	Were patients sufficiently homogenous with respect to prognostic risk?
	Were unbiased criteria used to detect the outcome in all patients?
	Was follow-up rate adequate?

review on therapy, the validity criteria should at least include randomization and adequacy of allocation concealment (see Table 6.1). In general, included studies that are of weak quality tend to overestimate the effectiveness of an intervention[5].

Tackle Box 6.1 How to interpret forest plots

Instructions: The balloons below label the most important parts of the forest plot. Go through these labels and familiarize yourself with the anatomy of the graph. Once you feel sufficiently familiar with the anatomy, go through the notes below on what the forest plot can signify.

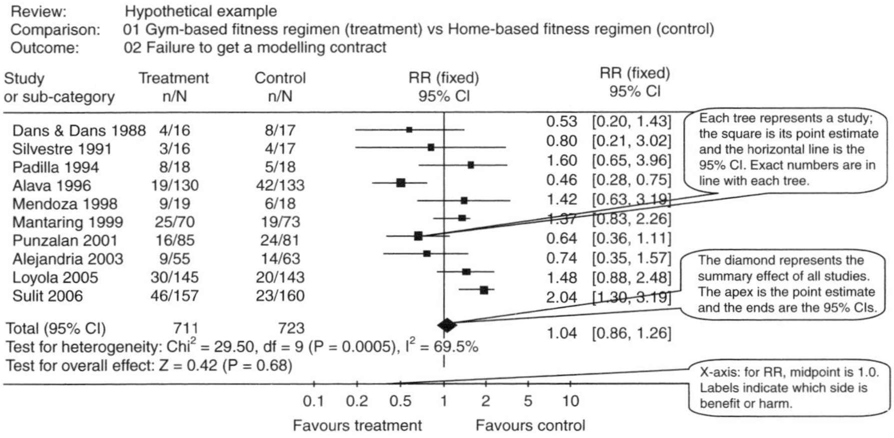

Review: Hypothetical example
Comparison: 01 Gym-based fitness regimen (treatment) vs Home-based fitness regimen (control)
Outcome: 02 Failure to get a modelling contract
Study or sub-category | Treatment n/N | Control n/N | RR (fixed) 95% CI | RR (fixed) 95% CI
Dans & Dans 1988 | 4/16 | 8/17 | 0.53 [0.20, 1.43]
Silvestre 1991 | 3/16 | 4/17 | 0.80 [0.21, 3.02]
Padilla 1994 | 8/18 | 5/18 | 1.60 [0.65, 3.96]
Alava 1996 | 19/130 | 42/133 | 0.46 [0.28, 0.75]
Mendoza 1998 | 9/19 | 6/18 | 1.42 [0.63, 3.19]
Mantaring 1999 | 25/70 | 19/73 | 1.37 [0.83, 2.26]
Punzalan 2001 | 16/85 | 24/81 | 0.64 [0.36, 1.11]
Alejandria 2003 | 9/55 | 14/63 | 0.74 [0.35, 1.57]
Loyola 2005 | 30/145 | 20/143 | 1.48 [0.88, 2.48]
Sulit 2006 | 46/157 | 23/160 | 2.04 [1.30, 3.19]
Total (95% CI) | 711 | 723 | 1.04 [0.86, 1.26]
Test for heterogeneity: Chi² = 29.50, df = 9 (P = 0.0005), I² = 69.5%
Test for overall effect: Z = 0.42 (P = 0.68)
0.1 0.2 0.5 1 2 5 10
Favours treatment
Favours control
Each tree represents a study; the square is its point estimate and the horizontal line is the 95% CI. Exact numbers are in line with each tree.
The diamond represents the summary effect of all studies. The apex is the point estimate and the ends are the 95% CIs.
X-axis: for RR, midpoint is 1.0. Labels indicate which side is benefit or harm.

Notes: A forest plot can tell us:

1. how many studies the review included: just count the number of trees!
2. which studies are the largest: the bigger the square in the middle, the bigger the study.
3. which studies had more outcome events: these have the narrowest 95% CI.
4. which studies showed statistically significant benefit (entire line is to the left of 1.0).
5. which studies showed statistically significant harm (entire line is to the right of 1.0).
6. which studies were inconclusive (line straddles 1.0 and extends far into either side).
7. which studies were inconclusive but showed a trend towards benefit (line is on the left, and barely touches 1.0).
8. which studies were inconclusive but showed a trend towards harm (line is on the right, and barely touches 1.0).
9. which studies show that the therapies are equal (line straddles 1.0 and doesn't go far to either side).
10. whether there are important differences (heterogeneity) between studies: if the lines hardly overlap, we should worry.

Notes 6 and 9 describe similar studies because they both straddle 1.0. However, they mean entirely different things. In note 6, the single study is *inconclusive* because confidence intervals are very wide. More studies need to be done. In note 9, the single study *is* conclusive that the two treatments are equal. The ends of the 95% CI are so close to 1 that they represent very small, unimportant harm and benefit. The situation in item 6 is sometimes referred to as 'absence of proof', while item 9 is referred to as 'proof of absence'.

Exercise: In the graph above, how many studies show (a) definite benefit, (b) definite harm, (c) inconclusive results and (d) equivalence of the two treatments?

Answers: (a) 1, (b) 1, (c) 8, (d) 0.

Question #4: Were the assessments of the studies reproducible?

Authors of systematic reviews decide on

(a) which studies to include;

(b) how valid these studies are; and

(c) what data to extract.

These may seem like objective tasks, but experienced reviewers will tell you that these are difficult judgments to make and are subject to human error. To ensure reproducible unbiased assessments in each of these tasks, there should be at least two independent reviewers. Also, check what steps the authors took to resolve disagreement. This is usually done by discussion or by calling in a third person.

6.3   Appraising the results

Question #1: What are the overall results of the review?

In a systematic review, a quantitative summary of the results is usually presented as a forest plot. If you are unfamiliar with the interpretation of forest plots, review Tackle Box 6.1 before proceeding.

Outcomes can be reported as dichotomous variables which have only two possible results, as we have demonstrated in Tackle Box 6.1 (i.e. given or not given a modeling contract). However, as described in Chapter 2, outcomes can also be reported as continuous variables that have a range of possible results (e.g. change in weight or blood pressure). When the outcomes are continuous, the difference between treatment and control groups

Review: Comparison of weight reduction programs
Comparison: Gym-based fitness regimen (treatment) vs. Home-based fitness regimen (control)
Outcome: Mean weight loss in lbs.

Study or sub-category	N	Control Mean (SD)	N	Treatment Mean (SD)	WMD (fixed) 95% CI
Dans & Dans 1988	16	15.25 (7.13)	17	13.81 (5.75)	
Silvestre 1991	16	18.34 (7.89)	17	16.54 (6.78)	
Padilla 1994	18	16.87 (4.77)	18	17.92 (5.23)	
Alava 1996	130	25.40 (9.30)	133	21.10 (8.20)	
Mendoza 1998	19	17.00 (2.08)	18	18.30 (2.34)	
Mantaring 1999	70	22.00 (12.00)	73	25.00 (9.00)	
Punzalan 2001	85	22.80 (16.70)	81	21.30 (14.10)	
Alejandria 2003	55	24.32 (8.66)	63	22.00 (9.35)	
Loyola 2005	145	23.00 (5.12)	143	26.23 (6.26)	
Sulit 2006	157	24.23 (3.00)	160	27.40 (4.60)	
Total (95% CI)	711		723		

Test for heterogeneity: Chi^2 = 59.29, df = 9 (P < 0.00001), I^2 = 84.8%
Test for overall effect: Z = 6.49 (P < 0.00001)

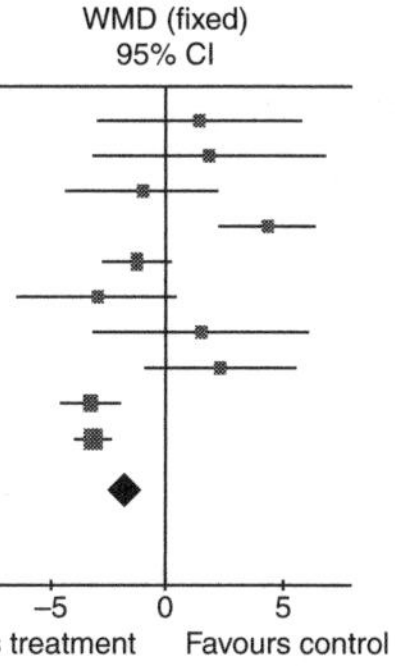

$$-5 \quad 0 \quad 5$$
Favours treatment   Favours control

WMD = weighted mean difference

Figure 6.1 Forest plot of a hypothetical systematic review evaluating a continuous outcome

can no longer be expressed as a relative risk reduction, absolute risk reduction or relative risk. Instead, the difference in outcome is simply expressed as the difference in means between treatment and control. Figure 6.1 illustrates a forest plot of hypothetical studies evaluating a continuous outcome.

Question #2: Were the results similar from study to study?

With a reasonably focused clinical question and appropriate inclusion and exclusion criteria, one would expect that the results would be similar from one study to another. However, this may not always be the case. Between studies, there may be slight variations in the characteristics of the population (P), the administration of the exposure (E) or the definition of the outcome (O).

Even when the PEOs are sufficiently similar, it is possible that the study methodologies used are slightly different (M). When such heterogeneity is present, reviewers are hesitant to perform a meta-analysis and estimate the average results. This is understandable as averages don't make sense unless we are averaging the same things. For example, a systematic review of mammographic screening for breast cancer would probably show no difference between screened and unscreened women if we analyse *all* age groups. Such a conclusion would be totally wrong and misleading. Screening is definitely beneficial among women aged 50 or more[6] and probably harmful among younger women[7].

To determine whether the results are similar enough to justify combining them, check whether the authors assessed for heterogeneity. There are two ways of assessing heterogeneity. One is by visual inspection of the forest plot to check if the trees from different studies overlap. This was discussed in Tackle Box 6.1. The second method is by performing statistical tests.

The chi-squared test is the most popular way of testing for heterogeneity. When the p value of the test is significant ($p < 0.10$), it is quite probable that differences exist among studies that cannot be attributed to chance alone. If you study the example in Tackle Box 6.1, you will see this test in the lower left hand of the sample forest plot.

Another statistical measure of heterogeneity is the I^2 statistic. While results of the chi-squared test indicate presence or absence of heterogeneity, the I^2 statistic provides information on the magnitude of heterogeneity. A value greater than 50% suggests substantial heterogeneity[8]. This value is seen next to the chi-squared test in Figure 6.1.

When studies are significantly heterogeneous, the authors should identify the sources of heterogeneity. Since differences in PEO or M are the common reasons for heterogeneity, dividing the studies into homogenous subgroups may minimize the problem. Another strategy would be to exclude apparent outlier studies and check if heterogeneity is corrected. This is referred to as a sensitivity analysis. When these subgroup analyses are not planned beforehand, their results should be viewed with caution. Too much exploration raises the possibility of accidental findings. If you torture the data enough, you might just get a confession!

Question #3: How precise were the results?

Because studies merely estimate the effectiveness of therapy or accuracy of tests, it may be unduly precise to express these estimates as exact values. For example, it may be misleading to conclude that 'warfarin reduces the risk of stroke in patients with atrial fibrillation by 79.0% (RRR)'. Such an estimate may sound too precise. It does not convey the uncertainty of the estimates. Therefore, researchers also express the treatment effect as an interval estimate which provides a range of possible values. Systematic reviews provide us point estimates and 95% CIs for individual studies (the lines in a forest plot) and, sometimes, for an overall estimate (the diamond at the bottom of a forest plot). As expected, the 95% CI around the summary value will always be narrower than the 95% CI around the individual studies. This gain in precision is the main reason we carry out systematic reviews at all.

6.4 Assessing applicability

Assessing the applicability of the results of a systematic review to your individual patient follows the same principles described in Chapters 2–5. Depending on whether you are appraising a systematic review on therapy, diagnosis, harm or prognosis, you can refer to the respective applicability sections of these chapters.

If the overall results of the review are not directly applicable to your patient population, do not despair. Valid subgroups may have been analysed that fit your patient's characteristics. As mentioned earlier, however, results derived from a subgroup analysis should be interpreted with caution. Criteria for determining whether the findings from subgroup analysis are credible include the following[9, 10].

1. The subgroup analysis should be pre-planned.

2. There shouldn't be too many subgroup analyses.

3. Subgroup differences, if found, should be seen consistently in different studies.

4. Subgroup differences, if found, should be biologically plausible.

When there are too many subgroup analyses and when many of them are unplanned, beware! Again too much exploration can lead to accidental findings.

6.5   Individualizing the results

Application of the results to an individual patient or patient group depends on what type of research question the systematic review addresses. These are discussed in detail in the sections on individualization of Chapters 2–5. Table 6.2 summarizes recommendations from these chapters.

A note of caution when dealing with systematic reviews on therapy: the reported ARR and NNT is averaged, rather than individualized. Therefore, these numbers may not apply to specific patients that you see. You need to seek the summary RR or RRR then go through the calculations described in Tackle Box 2.4 to estimate patient-specific results.

Table 6.2 Information needed for individualization of results by type of research question

Type of research question	What you need from the patient	What you need from the study	The individualized statistic you derive
Therapy[a]	The baseline risk based on clinical characteristics	The relative risk (RR) or relative risk reduction (RRR)	The individualized absolute risk reduction (ARR) or individualized number needed to treat (NNT)
Diagnosis[b]	Pre-test probability	Likelihood Ratio for a test result	The post-test probability of disease
Harm[c]	Baseline risk	Odds Ratio or Relative Risk	The individualized absolute risk increase (ARI) or number needed to harm (NNH)
Prognosis[d]	Baseline characteristics	Event rate or event-free survival	The patient-specific probability of developing complications

[a] Tackle Box 2.2
[b] Tackle Boxes 3.3 and 3.4
[c] Tackle Box 4.3
[d] Section 5.5

6.6 Summary

Systematic reviews usually address questions on therapy; however, they occasionally address questions on diagnosis, harm and prognosis. Begin evaluation of a systematic review by ensuring that it provides a direct enough answer to the focused and sensible question that you ask. If so, appraise validity, ensuring the process of study inclusion was both thorough and objective. Appraisal of results will entail understanding forest plots. Aside from the magnitude of the overall effect and the 95% CIs, these graphs also tell us if the results were similar from study to study. Assessment of applicability and individualization of results will depend on the nature of the research question.

References

[1] Chalmers I and Altman D (eds.) 1995. *Systematic Reviews*. BMJ Publishing Group: London.

[2] Egger M, Davey Smith G and Rourke K. 2001. Rationale, potentials and promise of systematic reviews. In: *Systematic Reviews in Health Care: Meta-analysis in Context*. Second Edition. BMJ Publishing Group: London.

[3] Egger M and Davey Smith G. 1998. Bias in location and selection of studies. *British Medical Journal*. **316**: 61–66.

[4] Krleža-Jeri K. 2005. Clinical trial registration: The differing views of industry, the WHO, and the Ottawa Group. *PLoS Medicine*. **2**(11): e378.

[5] Oxman A, Guyatt G, Cook D and Montori V. 2002. Summarizing the evidence. *In* Guyatt G, Drummond R (eds.) *Users' Guides to the Medical Literature*. American Medical Association Press: USA.

[6] Nystrom L, Rutqvist LE, Wall S, Lindgren A, Lindqvist M, Ryden S Andersson I, Bjurstam N, Fagerberg G, Frisell J and Tabár L. 1993. Breast cancer screening with mammography: An overview of Swedish randomized trials. *Lancet*. **341**: 973–978.

[7] Gotzsche PC and Nielsen M. 2006. Screening for breast cancer with mammography. *Cochrane Database of Systematic Reviews*. 4(CD001877). DOI: 10.1002/14651858.CD001877.pub2.

[8] Clarke M and Oxman AD. (eds.) 2003. Cochrane Reviewers Handbook 4.2.0 [updated March 2003]. *In* The Cochrane Library, Issue 2. Update Software: Oxford.

[9] Fletcher RH and Fletcher SW. 2005. *Clinical Epidemiology: The Essentials.* Fourth edition. Lippincott Williams & Wilkins: Maryland, USA.

[10] Oxman AD and Guyatt GH. 1992. A consumer's guide to subgroup analyses. *Annals of Internal Medicine.* **116**: 78–84.

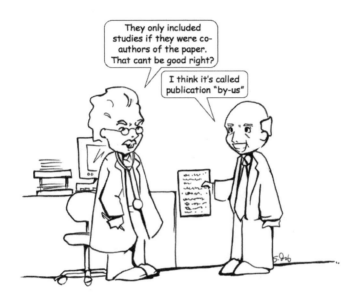

7

Literature Searches

Antonio L. Dans, Leonila F. Dans, Maria Asuncion A. Silvestre

If you were born in the 1950s or earlier, then you are probably old enough to remember what a pain it was to have to search the medical literature. The Index Medicus was the nightmare of every medical student. Sleep-deprived and bleary-eyed, students in medical libraries would hunch over endless rows of thick books that must have weighed tons when put together, to find that one elusive article that they needed. In fact, searching was such a pain then, that a journal search became a popular, sadistic form of punishment in medical schools. 'Don't be late for class or off you go to the dungeons of Index Medicus!' was the threat, accompanied by a crash of thunder in the background.

Fortunately, information access has evolved so much in the past two decades, that today we are able to search the entire Index Medicus at the click of a mouse! This is possible due to the fact that almost all databases of scientific publications are now available in electronic format. This development has cast manual searches into the depths of antiquity, but it has also raised new

Painless Evidence-Based Medicine   Antonio L. Dans, Leonila F. Dans and Maria Asuncion A. Silvestre
© 2008 John Wiley & Sons, Ltd

expectations from healthcare providers all over the world. Today, new (and not so new) generations of practitioners are expected to have skills for conducting thorough and efficient searches of the electronic medical literature.

7.1   What are electronic databases?

An electronic literature database can be likened to a file composed of several index cards. Each index card represents a published article, containing structured information such as its TITLE, the AUTHORS, the SOURCE, the ABSTRACT, KEYWORDS and other important information. In computer jargon, each index card is referred to as a RECORD, each piece of structured information is referred to as a FIELD and the entire conglomerate of index cards is referred to as the DATABASE. These relationships are illustrated in Figure 7.1.

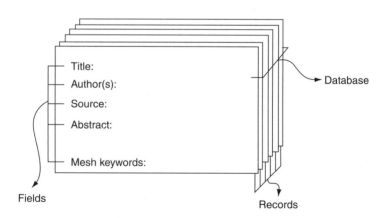

Figure 7.1   Components of an electronic database of medical literature

Each record represents an article containing structured information (fields) such as the author, source and abstract. A collection of records with structured information is called a database.

Numerous electronic databases of medical literature have emerged in recent years. The most popular (and the largest) is MEDLINE, which is managed by the US National Library of Medicine. As of July 2007, it contained 15 million articles from 5000 medical journals published in over 70 countries around the world. As many as 2000–4000 articles are indexed every working day[1]. EMBASE is another popular database, which indexes 375 000 articles a year from 3500 journals[2]. The Cumulative Index to Nursing & Allied Health Literature (CINAHL) Database stores articles from 2593 journals from various healthcare professions[3]. The Cochrane Central Register of Controlled Trials (CCRCT) has over 300 000 bibliographic references to controlled trials in health care. This database is an amalgamation of various sources[4]. Numerous other databases are available in various fields of the healthcare profession.

7.2   The language of electronic databases

Searching electronic databases requires a thorough understanding of Boolean language. This is not some ancient tongue unearthed from an advanced civilization which has been buried for centuries. On the contrary, Boolean language is very simple. It has just a handful of words, the usage of which you probably learned in elementary school. The best way to review Boolean syntax is by using the Venn diagram. Go through Tackle Box 7.1 to review the basic concepts. If you have children of school age, now would be a good time to ask for their help.

Tackle Box 7.1   The Venn diagram and Boolean language

Instruction: The Venn diagram below depicts three sets of numbers defined by the circles A, B and C. The numbers within each set are referred to as elements. In an electronic database of medical literature, the numbers represent various articles and the sets are key words or concepts that define these articles. Go through the description of Boolean language below, to understand how electronic databases work.

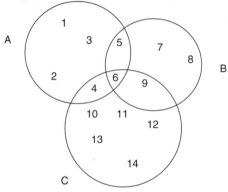

Boolean logic can be used to identify specific elements in this diagram. This is achieved using the connectives AND or OR. For example, the **union** of sets A and B can be expressed in Boolean language as A OR B. In the diagram, this would be represented by elements 1–9. Similarly, the **intersect** of sets A and B can be expressed as A AND B. In the diagram, this would be represented by elements 5 and 6. Note that unions (expressed by OR) tend to increase the number of elements included, while intersects (expressed by AND) tend to do the opposite. To make things more exciting, brackets can help us use unions and intersects in the same expression. Traditionally, operations with brackets are performed first. For example, to understand the expression (A AND C) OR B, first identify a new set defined by the intersect of A AND C. Complete the statement by getting the union of that new set with B. This whole statement would now refer to elements 4–9.

Exercise: Which elements do the following phrases refer to? a) B AND C; b) A AND B AND C; c) B OR C; d) A AND (B OR C).

Answers: (a) 6, 9; (b) 6 only; c) 4–14; (d) 4, 5, 6.

If you understand Boolean language and the difference between the connectives AND and OR, then you are ready to conduct an electronic search. While we refer to PubMed often in this discussion (because it is free online and accessible to all), the four steps we describe are also applicable to most other literature databases.

Step 1: Identify the concepts in your focused clinical question (P, E, O and M)

We have extensively discussed the components of a focused clinical question in previous chapters. P refers to the population of interest, E to the exposure being evaluated and O to the outcomes expected. If a clinical question is focused and well stated, it can often be clearly categorized into a quest for articles on therapy, diagnosis, harm or prognosis. The advantage of this association is that we can now link the focused question with specific study designs, using so-called methodological filters (M). For example, not only can we search for articles on treatment of osteoporosis (P) using bisphosphonates (E) to prevent fractures (O), but we can also narrow our search so that we only get randomized controlled trials (M)! A powerful feature of electronic databases is the ability to make the computer carry out some of the critical appraisal. Table 7.1 lists method filters you may want to use for various types of articles.

Step 2: Prioritize the concepts from most to least important

This is the tricky part of literature searches. Each concept in your question represents a set in the Venn diagram. If you intersect all these sets straight away, you may end up with nothing! The plan is therefore to intersect the concepts one at a time, until

Table 7.1 Method filters for various types of focused clinical questions

Type of question	Generic format	Method filter
Therapy	Among P, how effective is E in preventing O?	Systematic reviews or meta-analyses, RCTs, cohorts, case-control studies, case series or case reports
Diagnosis	Among P, how accurate is E in diagnosing O?	Studies that report 'sensitivity and specificity' or 'likelihood ratios', systematic reviews or meta-analyses
Harm	Among P, how much does E contribute to the causation of O?	Systematic reviews or meta-analyses, RCTs, cohorts, case-control studies, case series or case reports
Prognosis	Among P, by how much does E increase the risk of O?	Cohorts studies or systematic reviews or meta-analyses

Note: P = the population of interest (usually characterized by a disease or condition); E = the exposure being evaluated (either a treatment, a test, a harmful exposure or a prognostic factor); O = the outcome expected (a disease, complication or some measure of health).

you reach a manageable number of articles. Before you can do this, however, you need to decide which concept to search first (the most important) and which one to search last (the least important).

Which one is the most important? Ask yourself this: if you were allowed only one term to search, which concept would you search for? Consider the earlier example: among patients with osteoporosis (P) how effective are bisphosphonates (E) in preventing fractures (O)? Let's say you're interested in finding systematic reviews (M).

In this situation, which concept would you search first – P, E, O or M? If you search for articles on 'fractures' (O), you would be in trouble. There would be too many! The same would be true if you search for 'systematic reviews' (M). If you search for articles on 'osteoporosis' (P), you would pick up fewer articles but a lot would be on the use of other drugs such as calcium and vitamin D. However, if you search for articles on 'bisphosphonates' (E), they are likely to also be on osteoporosis and fracture prevention. Thus, the term bisphosphonates would be a reasonable start for this search, because it would yield the most useful set of articles.

If you search for articles on bisphosphonates and still get too many of them, then you need to try and narrow the search. Choosing the next best concept to search follows the same process. If you could intersect the first concept with just one other concept, which one would it be? Intersecting bisphosphonates with osteoporosis might yield a lot of articles you don't need such as cohort studies and practice guidelines, or even prevalence studies and letters to the editor. The same would be true if you intersect bisphosphonates with fractures. If you intersect bisphosphonates with systematic reviews, however, you are likely to get the most relevant yield. Systematic reviews on bisphosphonates (M and E) will most probably be about osteoporosis (P) and fractures (O).

If intersecting the first two concepts yields too many articles, then you need to choose a third. Again you ask: if you could intersect the first two concepts with just one other concept, which one would it be? In the example, adding fractures (O) as the third concept would filter out some studies (but not all) that just monitor effect on bone mass density (a mechanistic endpoint) and not fractures (a clinical endpoint). 'Fractures' would therefore be a reasonable third option. If you still get too many, then the fourth option is the only one left: osteoporosis (P).

Table 7.2 summarizes how this process of prioritization might be used for certain examples, including our bisphosphonate

Table 7.2 Examples of clinical questions, concepts and how they may be prioritized

Focused clinical question	Identified concepts	Rank*
Among patients with osteoporosis, how effective are bisphosphonates in preventing fractures?	P = patients with osteoporosis E = bisphosphonates O = fractures M = systematic reviews	4 1 3 2
Among patients with diabetes, how effective are sulfonylureas in preventing usual complications?	P = patients with diabetes E = sulfonylureas O = usual complications M = systematic reviews or RCTs	x 1 3 2
Among patients presenting with acute chest pain, how accurate is serum troponin-I determination in diagnosing acute myocardial infarction?	P = patients with acute chest pain E = serum troponin-I determination O = acute myocardial infarction M = studies that report sensitivity, specificity, or likelihood ratios	x 1 x 2

* Note: 1 = most important; 4 = least important; x = probably an unnecessary concept

example. As can be seen from these examples, prioritization can sometimes lead to the conclusions that some concepts are unnecessary. When searching for articles on sulfonylureas (P), for example, it is probably unnecessary to specify diabetes (P) as sulfonylureas are almost exclusively used for diabetes. Similarly, when searching for articles on serum troponin-I determination, it is probably unnecessary to specify P and O, because the test is specifically carried out to diagnose MI in patients with chest pain.

In our experience, the process of prioritization is extremely important but often neglected. Spend time to think through this prioritization step regularly so that it becomes intuitive. There are several advantages of making this a habit.

1. If searching priority concepts yields very few articles, then we don't need to use the lower priority concepts. This saves time.

2. We can also save time by skipping concepts that would not have improved our yield.

3. We avoid missing important articles because of mindless intersections.

Step 3: (a) Expand and (b) intersect each concept sequentially, until you obtain a manageable number of articles.

The previous two steps can be considered without even touching a computer key. These two steps represent the planning process before final implementation. Steps 3a and 3b comprise the bulk of the actual search. 'Expanding' a concept means trying to ensure that we account for different synonyms as well as different spellings. 'Intersecting' a concept means adding criteria to our search so that we limit it to only the articles that answer our focused question. To use the Venn diagram analogy, when we expand a concept we are trying to make our sets (represented by circles) as big as possible. We cast a wide net so that we include all the relevant articles in the concept. We then intersect these large circles, to get to the few articles that address all four components of our focused question. The cycle of expansion-intersection should be completed one concept at a time, using the sequence of priorities that you planned in Step 2.

To explore the intricacies of the expansion-intersection cycle, let's use the earlier example where we asked:

- Among patients with osteoporosis (P, 4th priority);

- how effective are bisphosphonates (E, 1st priority);

- in preventing fractures? (O, 3rd priority).

- We were looking for systematic reviews...(M, 2nd priority)

While reading the subsequent sections of this chapter, it is recommended that you be in front of a computer connected to your favourite electronic database of medical literature. We recommend PubMed (of the US National Library of Medicine and the US National Institutes of Health) at www.pubmed.com as it offers MEDLINE for free and has many neat features that make searching easy. If you aren't sure how to log on, you probably need someone beside you to provide guidance. Your best chance is anyone born in the 1970s or later. Figure 7.2 shows the home page of PubMed and its five main features which are useful for Step 3.

Step 3a: Expanding concepts

Expanding a concept using free text searches Start by looking for the search box of the database you use. Type the concept 'bisphosphonate', press the enter key, and *Voila*, . . . you have done a free text search! This is called a free text search not because it's free, but because it searches for words used freely by the authors in the title or abstract. Because the authors are not bound by conventions in spelling or terminology, they can use terms in any way they want. This is difficulty with the free text search strategy: the same concept can be referred to in different ways by different authors. 'Bisphosphonate' for example, may also

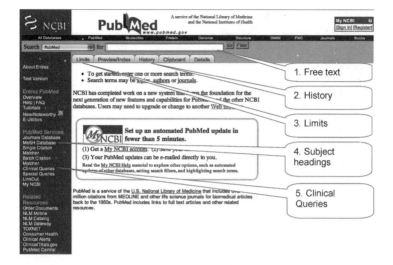

Figure 7.2 The main features of PubMed: (1) free text search; (2) search history; (3) search filters; (4) standardized terms for article classification and (5) search filters for articles on therapy, diagnosis, harm or prognosis

be referred to as '*bi*phosphonate'. To account for this, a better strategy would be to search for the union of the two terms, that is 'bisphosphonate OR biphosphonate'. Better yet, to account for plural forms of these words, we can type 'biphosphonate OR biphosphonates OR bisphosphonate OR bisphosphonates'. Try typing this in the search box to see that you do get a larger number of articles.

This is easy enough in our example but what if you have say, 20 synonyms and variations in spelling? Some electronic databases offer useful tricks to simplify the task.

1. History functions: Many electronic databases have a 'history' function which displays a numbered history of terms that you recently searched. Figure 7.3 shows a search for four spelling variations of bisphosphonates. Users can obtain the unions of

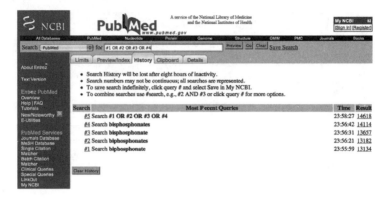

Figure 7.3 PubMed history feature, enabling previous searches to be combined

previous searches by typing their numbers in the sequence, instead of the terms themselves, e.g. '#1 OR #2 OR #3 OR #4'. Note that the union yields more articles than any of the four terms alone.

2. Truncations: Some words have the same roots, with variations primarily occurring in the suffix. In PubMed, the asterisk symbol (*) can be used at the end of root words so that all variations in suffix are captured. For example, try typing 'osteoporo*' in the search box. This will yield articles that use words beginning with 'osteoporo' such as osteoporotic and osteoporosis.

3. Phrase recognition: Sometimes a short phrase is one of the synonyms of a concept. For example, meta-analysis may also be referred to by the phrase *systematic review*. Electronic databases vary in how they search for phrases. Some look for an exact match but more advanced ones will automatically seek variations in word order and spelling. If you are sure about the phraseology of your search term however, it is best to enclose it

in quotation marks so that the database seeks an exact match. If you are not sure, entering the phrase without quotation marks may be your best option.

Expanding a concept using subject heading searches A more efficient way of solving the problem of non-uniform terminology is to use a standardized dictionary of medical terms to classify articles. MEDLINE uses a dictionary called MeSH (Medical Subject Headings). A similar dictionary called EMTREE is used by EMBASE. CINAHL also uses its own 'tree'. People entering articles into these databases continually check the dictionaries so they can classify articles in a standard way, regardless of the terms used by the authors.

Subject headings are very useful, because they obviate the need to create long lists of synonyms. Another advantage arises from the arrangement of the terms in hierarchal form, with trunks, branches, twigs and leaves. For example, Figure 7.4 below is from the MeSH tree of PubMed. It shows that 'female athlete triad syndrome' and 'osteoporosis, postmenopausal' are under

<u>All MeSH Categories</u>
    <u>Diseases Category</u>
        <u>Musculoskeletal Diseases</u>
            <u>Bone Diseases</u>
                Bone Diseases, Metabolic
                    <u>Bone Demineralization, Pathologic</u>
                        <u>Decalcification, Pathologic</u>
                    <u>Mucolipidoses</u>
                    <u>Osteomalacia</u>
                    <u>Osteoporosis</u>
                        <u>Female Athlete Triad Syndrome</u>
                        <u>Osteoporosis, Postmenopausal</u>
                  <u>Pseudohypoparathyroidism</u>
                    <u>Pseudopseudohypoparathyroidism</u>
                  <u>Renal Osteodystrophy</u>
                  <u>Rickets</u>
                    <u>Hypophosphatemic Rickets, X-Linked Dominant</u>
                    <u>Renal Osteodystrophy</u>

Figure 7.4 PubMed screen, displaying a portion of the MeSH tree

'osteoporosis', which is under 'bone diseases, metabolic', which in turn is under 'bone diseases'. Clicking on any branch in this tree will automatically search the twigs and leaves attached to it, again obviating the need for multiple terms and entries. In PubMed, this feature is called the 'explode' function. Don't take this literally; you don't have to run to your nearest bomb shelter. It is a default feature so all you need to do is click a term in the hierarchy and all sub-entries are searched automatically. Explode is especially useful when you are interested in a class of drugs, because then you don't need to enter the individual names.

Now try PubMed's MeSH tree on your sample problem. (You can access MeSH by clicking on the MeSH button in the left-hand column of any PubMed page.) As the screen shot in Figure 7.5 shows, if you enter the word 'bisphosphonates' in the search box, the MeSH synonym that will come up is 'diphosphonates'. We didn't know of this synonym, and therefore missed it altogether in our free text search! As it turns out, it is the standard term adopted by MeSH.

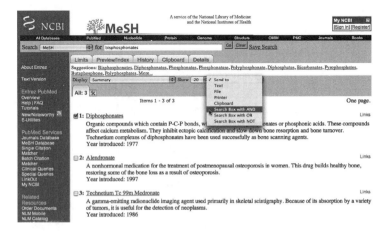

Figure 7.5 How a chosen MeSH term is used to search PubMed

Once a subject heading is chosen from the MeSH dictionary, there must be a mechanism to go back to the main database to actually search for articles on that subject. In PubMed, this is initiated by checking the tick box beside the term (e.g. diphosphonates), then clicking the 'send to search box' function. From the search box, PubMed can now be searched for relevant articles.

Figure 7.6 compares the search yield with MeSH (13 084 articles) and the search yield with the free text strategy that we used earlier (14 618). The difference is easily explained. Free text lists articles with the terms searched, even if they are not the main topic of the articles. MeSH only lists articles if the term searched is a key concept in that article. Most of the time therefore, MeSH will give you a better yield in terms of relevance. Researchers are often pressed to be very thorough in their searches. A trick we sometimes use is to search for the union of a free text and a subject heading. In this example, it would be stated as '#5 OR #7'.

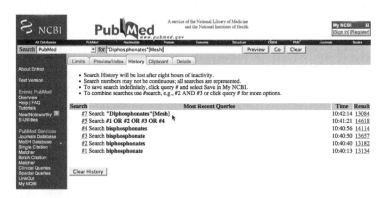

Figure 7.6 Use of PubMed history function to compare yield from a free text search (#5) and a MeSH search (#7)

Special strategies for expanding method searches Free text and subject headings may also be used to expand the method filters (M) identified in Table 7.2. 'Meta-analysis' can be a free text search, for example, and can also be found as a MeSH term. In addition however, some advanced electronic databases provide special tools to augment these two strategies. PubMed, for instance, has two features that we find very useful.

1. Limits: This feature provides a table with checkboxes for Publication types, such as randomized controlled trials, reviews or clinical practice guidelines.
   Tip: You need to keep track of whether you have the Limits function 'on' or 'off'. Forgetting to turn it off when you no longer need it is a common source of search errors.

2. Clinical Queries: PubMed lists this function in the blue margin on the left side of the PubMed screen. This feature contains pre-tested combinations of MeSH and free text strategies to search for certain study types. Users can actually select if they want to search for articles on therapy, diagnosis, prognosis or harm. In addition, they can select if they want a sensitive search (nothing missed, but many non-relevant articles) or a specific search (mostly relevant articles but some may be missed).
   Tip: If you're in a hurry, this might be a good choice of search strategy.

Step 3b: Intersecting concepts

By accessing many synonyms in step 3a, we are assuring the retrieval of all relevant articles (obtaining large Boolean sets). We face the danger, however, of retrieving thousands of articles, most of which we might not even need. Thus, a corollary strategy during the actual search is to narrow the yield by a sequential intersection of the concepts that were previously expanded. The number of concepts combined will depend on the yield at each step. Obviously, when the first step yields just a handful articles, it would be futile to proceed with additional combinations.

For the example on osteoporosis, whether we use the free text search for synonyms of bisphosphonates, the MeSH search using diphosphonates or the union of both, the yield will be around 14 000 articles. This is certainly not a manageable number; who, in their right mind, would want to read 14 000 titles and abstracts? We therefore need to intersect this concept with our second choice: a method filter. To do this, we can click the Limits function, click on Publication types, then 'meta-analysis'. In Figure 7.7 below, we see a yield of only 37! Another strategy would be to click 'Clinical Queries' to search for systematic reviews. To do this, simply type the history number of our Mesh search for diphosphonates, as shown in Figure 7.7. Click 'Go' and lo and behold: we have found 38 articles! Now this may not seem like a big difference in this example, but in many instances, the difference in yield can be quite large. In our experience, Clinical Queries have been extremely useful in simplifying our search for articles.

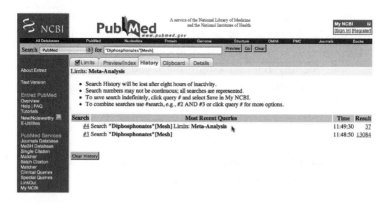

Figure 7.7 Using PubMed Limits function to search for certain study types (in this case a meta-analysis)

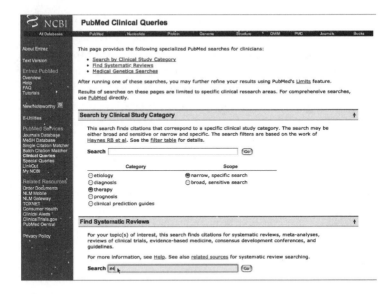

Figure 7.8 PubMed Clinical Queries feature, allowing articles to be searched for by type

Depending on how much time you have, running through the titles and abstracts of 37 or 38 articles may be considered manageable. If this is the case, you can now stop and just scan the titles for any relevant citations. If you don't have a lot of time, you will have to expand the next concept ('fractures') and intersect it with the first two concepts.

Step 4: Examine the yield for mishits and misses and revise the search if necessary

'Mishits' are articles yielded by our search that aren't relevant to our needs. 'Misses' are articles relevant to our search that our strategy did not find. Mishits are easy to assess. All you need to do is read through the list of articles found. Misses on the other hand, are difficult to assess and constitute a more serious problem. You never really know that you may be missing articles, unless you have some already in mind that you know should have come up. Figure 7.9 below shows that there were 37 articles yielded by our strategy. The first two seem to be mishits, but that's fine as long as we don't miss the good stuff. The third article seems to be relevant.

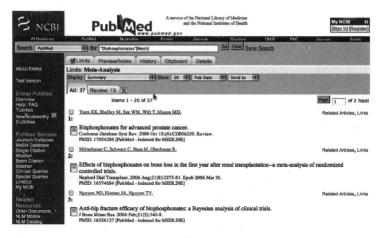

Figure 7.9 The different articles found by our search strategy

When we do find them, mishits are also easier to handle. When there are too many mishits, what can we do? We can:

1. expand and intersect more concepts; or

2. insert more stringent method filters (e.g. expand and intersect 'placebo' to obtain only studies with a placebo control group).

When there are too many misses (low yield), we can:

1. reduce the number of concepts;

2. use less stringent method filters; or

3. look for more synonyms by going through the initial yield.

If you were using free text, try expanding with MeSH. If you were using MeSH, try expanding with free text, or use the union of MeSH and free text searches.

7.3 Summary

A proper search begins with steps that don't even require a computer: identification of concepts (Step 1) and prioritization according to importance (Step 2). The search proper involves a cycle of concept expansion (Step 3a) and intersection (Step 3b), until a manageable (readable) number of articles are located. Examining the yield for mishits and misses can lead to an improvement of the strategy (Step 4).

Skill in literature searching is very empowering. You can obtain information straight away, when you really need it. This chapter has provided a few general points to help you, but you must practice to master the skill. Make it a habit to spend a few minutes everyday to search for topics of interest and hone your skills. Remember, finding a relevant article doesn't necessarily mean that your search strategy was a good one. You can always find an article by luck! Lucky searches reinforce bad technique, so don't use the yield to assess adequacy of your strategy. Instead, concentrate on method to ensure that your searches are reliable.

References

[1] http://www.nlm.nih.gov/pubs/factsheets/medline.html
[2] http://info.embase.com/embase_com/about/index.shtml
[3] http://www.cinahl.com/library/library.htm
[4] http://www.mrw.interscience.wiley.com/cochrane/
    cochrane_clcentral_articles_fs.html

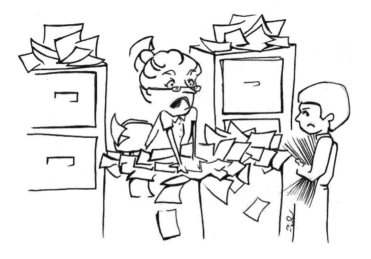

'You printed 5,275 abstracts? I asked you to search on global warming, I didn't ask you to cause it!'

Index

Painless Evidence-Based Medicine   Antonio L. Dans, Leonila F. Dans and Maria Asuncion A. Silvestre
© 2008 John Wiley & Sons, Ltd

Index compiled by Terry Halliday